Archetypal Healing through Fairy Stories and Myths

In this book, Victor MacGill uses the science of systems theory to explore the hidden meanings of fairytales and myths. He links the scientific with anthropological, mythological, psychological, and healing approaches to explore these stories and how they can be applied to emotional healing.

Throughout history, shared understandings of ourselves and our world have enabled us to cooperate. This book uses MacGill's 'dynamics of life' model to explore these foundational roles – such as the king, the warrior, the magician, the lover, and the dragon – and explains how these shared mental patterns within a culture create archetypes that inhabit our inner worlds and guide our lives and can reveal deeper aspects of human behaviour. These archetypes are reflected in fairy stories and myths recited around the fireside for millennia. The book presents examples from around the world – including the Greek tale of Perseus, traditional fairy stories such as Hansel and Gretel and Rapunzel, and Pacific myths – to highlight the hidden depths of meaning within these simple stories, which are usually relegated to children's bedtime. MacGill suggests that we can meet and interact with our inner kings and magicians and confront our own dragons through dreams, meditations, journalling, and much more, allowing us to heal our emotional and societal wounds.

With its interdisciplinary exploration of this topic and discussion of Jungian psychology, this book offers a unique resource for postgraduate researchers and other scholars, as well as psychoanalysts, psychotherapists, and coaches of all backgrounds.

Victor MacGill has 45 years' experience in various helping professions, including in community support roles, as a probation officer, and as a clinical social worker. He holds a PhD in systems theory from the University of the Sunshine Coast, Australia. He hosts workshops on mythology, archetypes, and systems theory.

Archetypal Healing through Fairy Stories and Myths

The Dragon is the Pathway to Peace

Victor MacGill

Routledge
Taylor & Francis Group
LONDON AND NEW YORK

Designed cover image: M J Steffans

First published 2026
by Routledge
4 Park Square, Milton Park, Abingdon, Oxon OX14 4RN

and by Routledge
605 Third Avenue, New York, NY 10158

Routledge is an imprint of the Taylor & Francis Group, an informa business

British Library Cataloguing-in-Publication Data
A catalogue record for this book is available from the British Library

Library of Congress Cataloging-in-Publication Data
Names: MacGill, Victor author
Title: Archetypal healing through fairy stories and myths :
the dragon is the pathway to peace / Victor MacGill.
Other titles: Dragon is the pathway to peace
Description: First edition. | New York, NY : Routledge, 2026. |
Includes bibliographical references and index. |
Identifiers: LCCN 2025053401 (print) | LCCN 2025053402 (ebook) |
ISBN 9781041146148 hbk | ISBN 9781041146070 pbk | ISBN 9781003675266 ebk
Subjects: LCSH: Fairy tales–Therapeutic use | Mythology–Therapeutic use | Healing |
System theory | LCGFT: Folk literature
Classification: LCC RC489.F3 .M335 2026 (print) | LCC RC489.F3 (ebook) |
DDC 616.89/16–dc23/eng/20260316
LC record available at https://lccn.loc.gov/2025053401
LC ebook record available at https://lccn.loc.gov/2025053402

ISBN: 9781041146148 (hbk)
ISBN: 9781041146070 (pbk)
ISBN: 9781003675266 (ebk)

DOI: 10.4324/9781003675266

Typeset in Garamond
by Newgen Publishing UK

Contents

Figures

Preface

Back in 1995, I published my first book, *When the Dragon Stirs: Healing Our Wounded Lives Through Fairy Stories, Myths and Legends* (MacGill, 1995). I walked through the world of archetypes and fairytales, and the wealth of knowledge that could be gained about our journey through life. While what I wrote is still relevant 30 years later, I have since learned so much more about who we are as human beings and how the powerful messages hidden in the simple stories that we tell our children can enhance our lives. It was time to return to the magical land of fairytales and write another book.

The intervening years have taken me to many places, both in the world and in my mind, which have taught me so much. In particular, I discovered the systems sciences, which provided a framework that connected the world of science to my spirituality, helping me to make sense of life's many paradoxes. Instead of pulling the world apart to see how it works, the systems sciences step back and explore the bigger picture. They look for relationships between the parts and explore the underlying patterns and processes that shape our lives. They clarify and make sense of the patterns behind the stories.

It turns out that the patterns described in the systems sciences and those described in fairytales and myths have the same basic underlying structures, albeit expressed in unique ways. Bringing the two together creates a powerful tool for delving into the depths of what it means to be human.

Telling stories is a core aspect of humanity. It is an essential way in which we make sense of and feel connected to the world we live in. Stories place us in a time and a place where events unfold. They describe our lives, with our struggles and challenges, expressing the joy and pain of living. Some events unfold as we would wish; others do not. They help us to understand the mysteries of life, with its paradoxes and trade-offs. Stories bring us together to realise our shared humanity and suggest ways to create better futures.

These stories emerged many centuries ago. Each generation retold them in ways that made sense to them and then added their own embellishments, building layer upon layer of wisdom to create a majestic tapestry of connectedness. The cultures handed down from our ancestors still live within us through our DNA and our stories. We are learning today how trauma travels through the generations to impact us at the physical level (van der Kolk, 2015). This is equally so at the other layers of our being. So much of what I have absorbed from the culture around me is helpful and guides my life well; other patterns are harmful and need to be left behind or reframed. Our cultural heritage has both enriched our lives and left us with wounds to heal.

My journey has taken me to great heights and great depths. This will also be true for you. I cannot take away the pain and suffering, but I offer you this journey of self-discovery and tools to help you on your way.

Take heart and be courageous. Start your journey to renew yourself as a wiser, more coherent being. Rather than conquering your life, you will learn to live with yourself and your life.

AI Use Statement

AI tools were used solely for research and editorial support during the development of this book. No AI-generated content was used in the writing of the manuscript.

References

MacGill, VRD (1995). *When the Dragon Stirs: Healing Our Wounded Lives through Fairy Stories, Myths and Legends*. DragonStirs Enterprises.

van der Kolk, B (2015). *The Body Keeps the Score: Brain, Mind and Body in the Healing of Trauma*. Penguin.

How to Use This Book

This book invites you into a deep journey — one that moves through myth, shadow, archetype, and the hidden landscapes of the psyche. It is not a book to be rushed. It is a companion for reflection, insight, and transformation. To help you navigate the material safely and meaningfully, I offer a few guiding principles.

1. Take your time
   The stories and frameworks in these pages work best when absorbed slowly. Pause often. Let images and ideas settle. Notice what stirs in you. This is not a linear textbook; it is a journey with its own rhythm.
2. Expect activation
   Archetypes, myths, and shadow material can awaken emotions, memories, or sensations you may not have expected. This is normal. It is also a sign that something important is moving. If you feel overwhelmed, pause. Ground yourself. Return when you feel ready.
3. Do not journey alone
   Some exercises — especially visualisations or shadow encounters — can bring unconscious material to the surface. If you choose to engage deeply, I recommend having a trusted friend, therapist, or support person available. Transformation is powerful, but it is safer when witnessed.
4. Use the tools gently
   The techniques in this book are invitations, not prescriptions. Choose what resonates. Leave what doesn't. You are not required to do every exercise, nor to push beyond your capacity. Your psyche knows the pace.
5. Honour your own meaning-making
   My interpretations of myths and archetypes are one possible lens. You may find different meanings emerging for you — follow them. Your inner world is the true authority here.

6. This book is not therapy
   While the material can be healing, it is not a substitute for professional support. If you are dealing with trauma, grief, or significant emotional distress, please seek the guidance of a qualified practitioner alongside your reading.
7. Hold the journey lightly
   You may find yourself returning to certain stories again and again. You may skip ahead. You may read a chapter and feel nothing, then feel everything weeks later. All of this is part of the process. Let the book meet you where you are.

Introduction

My journey of self-discovery began by exploring and understanding the archetypes within me and how they influence my life. This has been an ongoing quest for many decades. My understanding has ripened with age.

Archetypes formed for our ancestors as they came to terms with the world in which they lived. There were ideas and images all about them that they needed to structure in a useful way. Once we came together in communities – talking, interacting, and forming shared understandings – the mapping of our cognitive world accelerated. Just as people need to speak the same language to understand each other, our whole culture and how we make sense of our world must be aligned with those with whom we share our world. Other animals, such as our primate relatives, generally only congregate in groups of 30–50, whereas humans can congregate in groups of thousands or even millions. We have evolved elaborate social rules and rituals, allowing us to live successfully in enormous cities; but this larger scale also brings challenges.

As our early ancestors gathered around the fire at night, gazing up at the stars, they forged bonds with one another. Their minds began to align, establishing a shared understanding of the world. This enabled them to exchange ideas and teach what they had learned. They formed meaningful concepts to make sense of what of they found in the world around them.

At the same time, they discovered that if they took on specialised roles, each applying their unique skills, their whole community could prosper. Some were better at gardening, others at caring for children. Others still were wiser and held the inherited knowledge of their way of life and the world about them. Yet others became warriors, guarding and protecting the people.

Everyone had to learn what each role entailed and what was expected of them in that role. They also needed to know how to behave in the presence of someone holding each role. Concepts and metaphors were passed down through the stories and songs of our ancestors, which exemplified how one should behave in their respective roles.

Other formulations of culture allowed those in the community to distinguish themselves from others and recognise their own. Each tribe developed unique styles of dress, dance, art, poetry, and much more, which became integral to the traditions that maintained their stability through the generations. These formulations of mental energy, clustered around social roles, became archetypes – rather like blueprints – which

DOI: 10.4324/9781003675266-1

guide our actions and help us to make sense of the behaviour of others. Each tribe formulated these in unique ways that aligned with their traditions.

Today, we live in very different times, but the basic archetypes remain relevant. Archetypes lie at the core of our being, but they evolve more slowly than the society to which they belong. We must continually reassess the archetypes that we use to ensure that they remain relevant. They are alive in us, and we can contact and work with them to find our pathway forward to create better futures for ourselves and our families.

The first part of this book (Chapters 1–6) introduces the central topic and reveals the foundational knowledge needed to explore the inner meanings of fairytales and myths. We investigate the work of Carl Jung and systems theory, which I call the science of connecting. Life is a dynamic process of connecting and disconnecting. We can use systems theory to track our evolution through levels of matter, life, mind, and culture. Archetypes arose as we developed human culture, but the nature of the lower levels constrained the form that the archetypes could take. We learn about the trade-offs that sit at the core of life, balancing order and chaos to form an 'Edge of Chaos' (Gleick, 1987; Prigogine & Stenger, 1984), where life can emerge and even take us to a higher level of being. Systems ideas link to Gregg Henriques' unified theory of knowledge, which frames evolutionary development through four phases. We cover fractals and how they link to archetypes. This takes us through to the dynamics of life model (MacGill, 2023), which pulls all the various threads together and enables us to find coherent meaning in shared stories. We also look at issues of sex and gender, cognitive mapping, and the role of metaphors.

The second part (Chapter 7) looks at five specific human archetypes that dwell within each of us and shape how we make sense of our world and interact meaningfully with each other. The king represents our authority, the warrior our courage, the magician our wisdom, and the lover our compassion. When these are out of balance, they generate the fifth archetype: the dragon.

With this wisdom integrated into a coherent framework, we embark on the third part (Chapters 8–12), which investigates myths and fairytales from around the world and reveals the keys to unlocking their secrets.

The book concludes by examines specific tools and techniques for working with archetypes to cultivate a more authentic, fulfilling life.

Welcome to the journey!

References

Gleick, J (1987). *Chaos: Making a New Science*. Abacus Books.

MacGill, VRD (2023). The Dynamics of Life Model. *Systems Research and Behavioral Sciences, 41*(2), 262–273.

Prigogine, I & Stenger, I (1984). *Order Out of Chaos*. New Science Library.

1 The Call to the Journey

Introduction

Everybody has a story and a journey to unfold. You are the hero of your own unique story. This is an exciting journey of discovery and revelation; but do not take it lightly. It is not for the fainthearted, for there are many pitfalls and perils along the way. There are many strange and often dangerous creatures to encounter, which will eventually be revealed as parts of ourselves.

First, we must make the necessary preparations, just as we would for any significant voyage. We must gather our vital possessions in our bag to sustain us on the journey. We must plan ahead so that we are ready for what we might encounter once we pass beyond the castle gates.

On a physical journey, we need clothes, food, and useful items. There may even be a magic potion or a special sword to help us overcome the challenges that await us. We must gather the precious knowledge, concepts, theories, and ideas that will support us on our quest.

Just as there are different stages in a journey that follow each other, this book has chapters that follow each other. They will enable us to explore archetypes from a variety of perspectives. We must first prepare for the journey by gathering the knowledge and concepts necessary to undertake it. We will learn about Carl Jung and Jungian psychology and link these ideas to the principles of the systems sciences, which reveal many of the underlying dynamics that create the cultures in which we live and the archetypes that we live by.

This will lead us to the hero's journey. We each live our own version of this story as we navigate our lives, meeting a wide range of characters along the way. Some will help and support us; others will try to stop us. We will face the dragons that oppose our forward movement. Underneath the dragon's roar is a call for healing. Those things that we least want to acknowledge as a part of ourselves are precisely the parts that we need to heal and develop.

Because our lives are not static, the archetypes within are not static either. As the challenges of our age change, the archetypes also change; but they change more slowly than the events of our lives, so we need to update them to be relevant to our age. Archetypes can help us to make sense of issues such as racism, sexism, and gender. Let us begin collecting the provisions for our journey that will be kept within our bag.

DOI: 10.4324/9781003675266-2

Carl Jung and Jungian Psychology

Our first precious possession comprises the ideas of Carl Jung and the Jungian psychologists. According to Jung, we divide our being into one part that is conscious and another that is unconscious (Jung, 2014). As a baby grows, they learn to distinguish themselves from the world around them. They have a body that moves in the world and a mind that makes sense of what arises as the body moves about. Our body has a finite amount of energy available (Feldman Barrett, 2017) so it economises on energy use by making certain processes unconscious. For example, we do not need to think about keeping our heart pumping or taking our next breath. It is all unconsciously controlled. Many functions of our mind are similarly unconscious. This leaves us free energy to focus consciously on those functions that require further attention.

The ego sits in the conscious mind, managing the border between the conscious and the unconscious. Within our unconscious mind lies the personal unconscious, which contains our emotions and experiences that occurred throughout our lives, which we could not manage at the time the events happened. Jung believed that other parts of our unconscious arose from our inherited past, which he referred to as the 'collective unconscious'. Archetypes dwell in the collective unconscious.

Jung wrote: 'Archetypes are universal, inborn models of people, behaviours, or personalities that play a role in influencing human behaviour. They are innate, hereditary, and universal, organising how we experience certain things throughout life' (Jung, 2014). Archetypes are, therefore, constellations of mind energy that have arisen as we interact together as communities and societies throughout history (Colman, 2008, 2011). Researchers in other disciplines have proposed psychic formations that resonate with the concept of archetypes. In the 1940s, Lorenz and Tinbergen (1951) described innate releasing mechanisms, suggesting a connection with archetypes in the biological realm. Charles Darwin (1859/1993) used the term 'archetype' to refer to stable psychic structures that natural selection could modify. Lakoff and Johnson (1980) spoke of archetypes as 'conceptual metaphors', which form a framework for understanding the world. Noam Chomsky (1965) contended that a universal grammar underlies all language. Christopher Alexander (1977) introduced the idea of recurring patterns in architecture.

Stevens (2006) writes of archetypes as having both a biological aspect and a mental aspect; as such, they arguably provide a solution to Descartes' mind-body problem. Descartes believed that the mind and body were separate, but Jung saw them as unified. Quantum physicist Wolfgang Pauli agreed with Jung, linking the mind-body problem to the wave-particle problem (Meier, 2001).

Jung proposed a *unus mundus*, a unified psychic world, which is the foundation of all mind. It is from this *unus mundus* that archetypes arise. The fact that everything arises from the one source links to Jung's ideas of synchronicity. If the universe is fractal (Mandelbrot, 1982), with each part connected to every other through the *unus mundus*, then we could expect an event in one part of the universe to have a symbolic reflection somewhere else. I remember coming home from my uncle's funeral and seeing a monarch butterfly land on my windscreen, which stayed there for some time. At another time, I had the clear feeling of a spirit passing, only to learn that an old friend had died at just that moment. These reflect some of the more esoteric ideas of Jung that some people might not be attracted to. If such an esoteric approach does not work for you, you can put it aside and still gain from the core of Jung's ideas.

We can only communicate when we have a shared way of making sense of the world that we live in. The colour red, or the concept of mother, must be sufficiently similar between people for them to be able to talk about it. Over thousands of years, these have become so deeply embedded within us that we do not usually notice them. All people are born with archetypes within them as part of their cultural heritage, which helps us to collaborate effectively through common understandings. Each culture expresses the inherent archetypes in a form that suits that culture and its nature.

Jung (2014) argued that cultural transmission was not adequate to explain the existence of archetypes as seen in myths around the world. There are similarities between cultures that have no connection, and archetypal symbols appear in the dreams and meditations of people with no understanding of the symbols or possible interpretations.

Jung was clear that there is an infinite number of archetypes, and that these are diverse and cannot be understood without taking their context into account. Archetypes overlap with each other and assume a life of their own, operating as complex adaptive systems (Miller & Page, 2007).

The Persona

Carl Jung distinguished three archetypes within all human beings at the level of the mind: the Self, the shadow, the anima, and the animus. Just as the various parts of the body interact and cooperate to act as one, the different parts of our mind interact and collaborate so that we can act in coherent ways. Jung also discussed the persona as linked to these archetypes; but the persona is a complex entity rather than an archetype, since it arises within each individual rather than being a universal, shared aspect of being. The persona is the mask that we wear between ourselves and the people of the outside world. The society that we live in is established around rules of what is appropriate and what is not. There are ideas we have that we would not feel safe to make public. We hide parts of ourselves from public view because we are concerned about how others would perceive them.

The Self

The Self is the whole mind, both conscious and unconscious. Jung uses a capital 'S' to distinguish this use of the Self from its more everyday usage. The Self comprises interacting parts that function as a whole. We will learn that this pattern of parts forming into wholes occurs within all complex systems, especially living or social systems. Jung talked about individuation – the process of becoming a complete individual. To achieve this, we must harmonise all the conflicting aspects of our being. To represent completeness, Jung often symbolised the Self as a circle, square, or mandala. Jung paradoxically writes of the Self as an archetype; while at the same time, it is the total of who we are individually.

In *Act and Image* (2021), Warren Colman argues that archetypes arose as symbolic images tied to our social interactions, often based on the material objects in our world. Women's clothing became associated with the concept of mother. Drawings on cave walls became images that stood for something in the real world. Our embodied actions shaped how we sensed and acted in our world. Of course, language also creates links between symbols and the real-world objects and events that we live through.

Colman also asks whether the Self is found or made. Is it something that is there unrealised, which we discover fully formed? Or does it not exist until we create it through our interactions with others? Colman seeks a middle path where both are true at once. Put another way: do I create my world or I am created by the world I live in? Both are true: we both create and are created. Perhaps the Self is like an acorn. It is not a tree – it is not even the blueprint of a tree; yet it shapes the possibilities of what the tree might become. These ideas fit comfortably with the concepts of systems theory that follow. Systems also look for the synthesis of the paradox rather than choosing one 'correct' answer.

To act effectively in the world, we must act quickly enough before the situation changes yet again and accurately enough to take us towards our goals and minimise the use of energy. We can only ever make our best guess, because we cannot know everything about ourselves and our world. We must make guesses and assumptions about ourselves and our world, which are sometimes incorrect. This creates tensions within the Self.

The Shadow

We form an internal map of ourselves in our psyche as best we can. It will always be incomplete, but we use this imperfect map to create a coherent sense of self. We can embrace some aspects of ourselves; but aspects that contradict our map cause dissonance, so we often conceal those parts by making them unconscious. Our persona hides what we do not want others to see and the personal unconscious hides what we are unwilling to know about ourselves.

The parts of ourselves that we are not happy to show to others, or even to ourselves, form the shadow. This holds all the repressed emotions held in our fears, desires, instincts, and shortcomings. We may think that we have rid ourselves of experiences that we have repressed, but they can re-emerge into consciousness when triggered by certain events. The shadow sabotages our efforts to act well in the world.

Anima and Animus

Jung further proposed that within the Self are the anima and animus (Stevens, 2001). The anima is the female part of the male psyche and the animus is the male part of the female psyche. Gender and gender roles were more rigid in Jung's time, but even he was very clear that he was referring to psychic energy qualities rather than simply genders. Perhaps this refers to the interplay of rationality and assertiveness, dancing together with compassion and caring. Life is full of seeming polarities that are more like continuums or complementary pairs. They influence and are influenced by each other. The anima and animus are not social creations arising from roles lived out, such as those of a king or warrior, but rather go much deeper to the core of who we are as humans – which means that they are far less malleable. These mind forces must be balanced within us if we are to become whole. Jung proposed that there is an anima in men and an animus in women. More modern Jungian writers, backed up by empirical studies, suggest that both men and women have both anima and animus (Stevens, 2006). This is particularly evident today, as we have a much broader view of how gender might be experienced, with gay and transgender people being more visible. Gender is more of a dynamic balance; so, like the tightrope walker, we constantly adjust our balance to remain within the constraints that bind us.

Further Jungian Concepts

Jung believed that our lives follow two stages. In the first stage of life, we build our ego, balancing the constraints within the psyche to develop a sense of ourselves that enables us to function adequately in the world. In the second part, we re-evaluate our lives and reintegrate ourselves to heal the wounds and imperfections that were created growing through the first stage. Erich Neumann proposed that the first stage can be divided into two parts (Stein, 2006). From birth to adolescence is the realm of the mother energy, often fulfilled by the actual mother. Especially early on, the child is fused with the mother and cannot recognise the boundary between them. In this period, the child is highly dependent on their carer and cannot survive alone. They live in a world of unconditional love and acceptance, where they are safe from the harsh realities of life.

From adolescence – particularly through the teenage years – the father energy takes over, often again embodied in the actual father. The father takes the child away from the protective world of the mother to learn the skills of independence and individuality, including the ability to live in a harsh, unforgiving world. The transition between the mother energy and the father energy is a slow one, rather than an abrupt change. Early in life, things such as potty training involve the father energy of doing something that the child does not want to do.

Male energy must separate the child from the mother. This can be experienced as abusive or violent – and sometimes it is; but the child must find the courage and fortitude to live in a competitive, combative world of winners and losers. James Hillman (1972) argues that narcissism reflects a failure of psychic separation from the archetypal mother, leaving the personality infused with omnipotence and entitlement and unable to tolerate frustration or otherness. Narcissists demand to be the centre of attention. They cannot brook being wrong or not getting their way, just like a child. They tend to employ manipulative tactics to achieve this. Hillman further suggests that borderline personalities are those stuck in this transition. When they do not get their way, they display the negative aspects of the father energy and can be violent.

In her book *Awakening the Heroes Within* (1991), Carol Pearson identified 12 archetypes out of the infinite range of possibilities that unfold from the three archetypes already mentioned:

- **Magician:** Transforms situations by shifting perception, insight, or energy, often acting as a catalyst for change.
- **Creator/artist:** The creator might be God or gods, but they create where there was nothing before.
- **Sage:** The sage manifests wisdom.
- **Innocent:** The innocent is often found early in life, before the world's hard lessons have set in.
- **Seeker:** Driven by curiosity and the desire to 'go where no one has gone before'.
- **Destroyer:** Challenges what no longer serves, breaks down what is stagnant, and clears the way for renewal.
- **Warrior:** Develops courage, discipline, and the capacity to face challenges.
- **Fool:** Pokes fun at the ruler if the ruler has gone off track.
- **Orphan:** Represents the ordinary person, often feeling like an outsider looking in. The orphan stands for our shared humanity.
- **Lover:** The lover has compassion. Male and female are united under this archetype.
- **Caregiver:** The nurturer and carer must care especially for the vulnerable.

These archetypes fit together as a complementary set, suggesting a wholeness when combined. They are mappings within the psyche of parts of our mind that often play out in society as social roles.

Many archetypes arose to encapsulate social roles. Initially, when there were few different social roles, there were not as many archetypes; but as the number of roles in society increased, so too did the number of archetypes. The focus of this book is on archetypes that have arisen from social roles. Other archetypes emerged as qualities of human life and behaviour, such as wisdom, love, and truth, or mother and father. Indeed, the number of potential archetypes is infinite, as Jung stated. Many archetypes overlap and blend into one another.

Jung mentioned the concept of 'The Third'. He proposed that in a couple relationship, an emergent symbolic form arises from the interactions between the two people (Colman, 2007). This fits comfortably with systems principles of emergence. It can be particularly useful if we tend to polarise viewpoints. All too often, either person in a relationship sees the other as the problem. In fact, it is often neither; instead, the conflict arises from the interactions between them.

Jung's last book was *Answer to Job* (2010). He explored the Book of Job, treating God as a mythological character. He found Job to be an upstanding, moral person who maintained his faith and honour. God, on the other hand, demanded loyalty and broke promises – all for a wager with the Devil.

Jung read this as a fundamental challenge of God, where God is called upon to take accountability for his actions. Jung suggests that the pain unfairly meted out to Job by God reveals a darker side to God. Being forced to see himself as he is, God is prompted to send Jesus Christ into the world to redeem mankind. Thus, God in man acknowledges his shadow side and heals the connection between God and man. Jung also saw a connection to the hidden feminine aspect of God in man.

Jean Knox (2012) has taken Jung's original ideas and reshaped them in line with findings from neurobiology and more modern techniques from working with clients to strengthen and improve the base of Jung's work. She notes that Jung's concepts have tended to be sidelined by other styles of psychology, even though many of them have been proven to be consistent with modern research (Roesler, 2024). Some Jungian scholars today suggest that archetypes are so deeply embedded as to be a part of our DNA (Rahman, 2025). Rather than seeing archetypes as innate images ready formed, she views them as a framework within the psyche, established by mental constraints, from which emergent properties arise that each culture fills with its own content.

Knox examines John Bowlby's work on attachment theory (Bowlby, 1983; Metcalf, 2010), which examines how a child bonds, or fails to bond, with the mother or primary carer and how that impacts their later life. Some children develop secure attachment styles; others are anxious, avoidant, or disorganised; and others still exhibit a mix of both. The story of the Lion King might be helpful for a disorganised child. The Snow Queen, Beauty and the Beast, and the Ugly Duckling might be beneficial stories for children with avoidant styles; while Hansel and Gretel, the Velveteen Rabbit, and the Tale of Peter Rabbit may be more suitable for children with an anxious style. Cinderella works well for securely attached children. Someone with an insecure attachment might repress archetypal patterns tied to dependency or intimacy. Therapy helps to identify and integrate these patterns.

Knox (2012) describes narrative as a tool that a baby learns by hearing stories such as fairytales to help make sense of cause and effect – how actions have consequences in the long term. The child learns to make sense of the events in their life coherently. They grow to understand that sometimes things come together magically, and sometimes life can be bitter and harsh. Knox notes that it is through narratives that we learn to reflect on the events of our lives, and on ourselves and others, enabling us to connect with others and build empathy.

Michael Fordham (1995) suggests that the processes of the development of the self as an individual are mirrored in how we form our social reality. Issues such as the failure to integrate the shadow might lead to political extremism in an individual or allow for the rise of a populist dictator within a society. Such a tyrant can tap into the shadow archetype within the collective unconscious and externalise their shadows into a scapegoat, creating a false sense of identity and avoiding the shadow.

The Systems Sciences

Our second magic ally in this journey is the systems sciences (Capra & Luisi, 2014), which I like to call the 'science of connecting'. Most scientific endeavours try to understand the world by taking it apart bit by bit until the pieces are small enough to understand. The problem with this approach is that it loses sight of the whole picture and of the relationships between the parts. We can dissect a rat and learn a great deal about how its body works, but that will never truly teach us about a living rat. We saw above that life is arranged so that parts come together to make wholes. Systems are interested in processes that happen over time as parts interact. The process tells a story. The concept of systems was only just emerging in Jung's time, but we know much more today, allowing for an interesting synthesis of Jungian ideas and systems principles. Life is the process of things coming together and then breaking apart again until the whole cycle starts again. We talk of systems sciences because, rather than one set of ideas, this is (ironically) a system of concepts and ideas that fit together to form a coherent, unified understanding of ourselves and the world that we live in.

The Breath of Life

Life breathes. There is a universal underlying flowing pattern of life. Life expands until it reaches a limit and then contracts, drawing in until it again reaches another limit, which brings it back to its initial state and starts a new cycle. Breathing in and breathing out, life maintains its dynamic flow, expanding and contracting at all scales of existence, from the tiniest amoeba to Gaia, our whole planet.

Our day expands in the morning light, then contracts back into darkness. The moon expands and contracts every month. Over our lifetime, we expand during our youth, mature as adults, and contract into old age. We grow, creating order in our lives to achieve things; but eventually chaos creeps in, breaking apart what has grown. Life arises from the dynamic tension of order and chaos, performing a delicate dance over and over (Gleick, 1987; Prigogine & Stenger, 1984). Taoism espouses the concept of yin and yang. Yang is the male, expansive, ordered force that builds things up in the universe. Yin is the female, chaotic force that breaks things down (Briggs & Peat, 1989). They are complementary, not opposites. There is always yang in the yin and yin

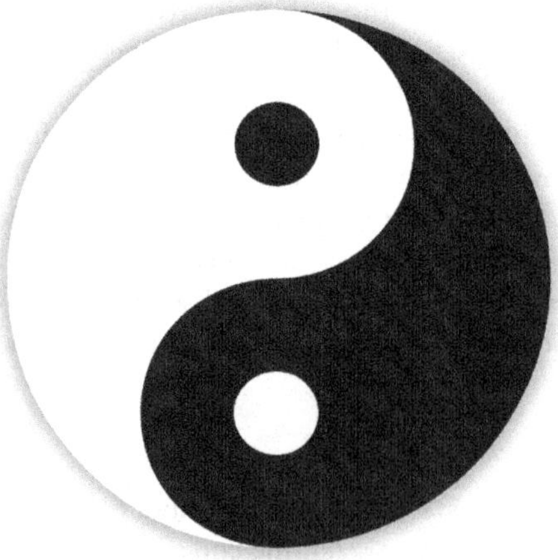

Figure 1.1 The yin-yang symbol.

Yang is white and yin is black. The two are complementary. Yin flows into yang and yang flows into yin. There is always yin in the yang and yang in the yin.

Source: Wikipedia Public Domain.

in the yang. Yang expands until it can expand no more and becomes yin. Yin contracts until it can contract no more and again becomes yang.

Life is all about separate parts coming together to cooperate because they can achieve more together than they can separately. Together, the interacting parts form a system. Two people working together can carry loads that neither could have lifted individually. The more people who work together, the greater the pool of knowledge, skills, and resources available. The more the system grows, the more it can grow. But systems cannot grow forever. The larger a system becomes, the more infrastructure it requires to support and control itself. There is always something that will end the expansion. The system starts to come apart and the parts that make it up become free to come together in new ways in a new cycle.

A system might be composed of atoms that form into molecules, molecules that form body cells, body cells that come together into body tissue, tissues that combine to form glands, and glands that develop into organs, which in turn form body systems such as the respiratory, skeletal, and nervous systems. These all come together as a whole human being. People come together to form communities, which in turn form cities, which ultimately form nations. We find systems of systems. Subsystems come together to form systems and the systems come together to form supersystems.

Holling and Gunderson (2002) devised a four-stage description of the life cycle that echoes life's connecting and disconnecting patterns. The 'Adaptive Cycle' starts with a growth or exploitation phase of expansion. This is followed by a conservation phase, during which growth slows. When the growth cannot continue, there is a descent into a release phase – what once came together now comes apart. The final reorganisation phase brings the system back to a new growth phase.

A company starts with just a few employees. It is flexible and adaptable, but not very strong or organised. As it grows, it adds more employees and thus requires a larger, more complex infrastructure to monitor all the processes and control how all the resources are used. As it continues to grow, the energy needed to power the infrastructure takes up a bigger percentage of the available energy. Rules become inflexible and the company becomes rigid. It becomes unable to adapt quickly to changing markets and starts to contract. It tries its best to hang on to its power, but inevitably, it starts to fall apart. As it fails, the seeds of a new cycle are sown. If the people running the business are alert and wise, they can bring the company through to a new cycle. If they cannot, the company will fail.

After a fire has destroyed all the old trees in a forest, the seeds that have fallen to the ground find space to start germinating and growing. A new generation of forest emerges and begins to grow. Over time, all the flora and fauna return. There is plenty of rain and sunlight for everything to grow. The forest becomes increasingly complex and interdependent. Certain species become dominant, making it difficult, if not impossible, for new species to take hold. Everything now competes for resources. All new life that arises must fit within the patterns and constraints that have been established. A forest will typically stay in this growth/conservation state for a long time – perhaps thousands of years; but eventually it will become too rigid, making it less resistant to outside perturbations. An external event – such as a flood, fire, or earthquake – can trigger the forest to enter the release phase, where everything comes apart. Connections and interdependencies fall apart. Seeds are shed, ready for the next cycle.

These cycles and patterns are all around us, so they inevitably become woven into the stories that we tell. Stories breathe: the characters expand and contract, connect and disconnect. They have a natural flow, like the tides of the sea.

As humans lived on the land, we began telling stories about ourselves and the places that we inhabited. We collected stories of heroes who did great things that deserved to be remembered. At times, these stories became embellished and refined into myths, making them easier to remember. Sometimes, men and women became immortalised as gods. At other times, whole new heroic figures were created through stories. A myth or fairytale can often reveal more about reality than a factual story.

Some stories better embodied these underlying life patterns and were told more often. Over time, they were self-selected as examples to live by. These simple stories, now often relegated to bedtime, capture the essence of what it means to be alive, as they describe the journey that we must all undertake through our lives, breathing in and out.

Our lifetime is a story of growing and expanding and then retreating until we can retreat no more. This describes the hero's journey, as told by Joseph Campbell (2012). Over millennia, humans have observed the patterns of our lives and noticed the journey from innocence and dependence to wisdom and co-creation. We begin our journey in innocence, where we are unable to meet our needs. Adults assume responsibility for their actions. We grow into adulthood, where we must take responsibility for our lives and make our way in the world. We must confront the harsh realities of the world and the consequences of our actions and inactions. We will all have times when our actions fall short. We try to maintain our ego self, but in the end, it becomes unsustainable. We must come to terms with our fallibility and descend into our dark night to face up to the harshness of our life and recognise how we have constructed our own reality, with all its pain and suffering. Then, having learned the lesson, we need to return to life and share what we have learned with others.

References

Alexander, C (1977). *A Pattern Language: Towns, Buildings, Construction.* Oxford University Press.

Bowlby, J (1983). *Attachment* (1st Edition). Perseus.

Briggs, J & Peat, FD (1989). *Turbulent Mirror: An Illustrated Guide to Chaos Theory and the Science of Wholeness.* Harper and Row Publishers.

Campbell, J (2012). *The Hero with a Thousand Faces: The Collected Works of Joseph Campbell.* New World Publishers.

Capra, F & Luisi, PL (2014). *The Systems View of Life: A Unifying Vision.* Cambridge University Press.

Chomsky, N (1965). *Aspects of the Theory of Syntax.* MIT Press.

Colman, W (2007). Symbolic Conceptions: The Idea of the Third. *Journal of Analytical Psychology, 52*(5), 565583.

Colman, W (2021). *Act and Image: The Emergence of Symbolic Imagination* (1st Edition). Routledge.

Darwin, C (1859/1993). *The Origin of Species: By Means of Natural Selection of the Preservation of Favoured Races in the Struggle for Life*. Random House.

Feldman Barrett, L (2017). *How Emotions are Made: The Secret Life of the Brain*. Pan Books.

Fordham, M (1995). *Explorations in the Self*. Karnak.

Gleick, J (1987). *Chaos: Making a New Science*. Abacus Books.

Gunderson, LH & Holling, CS (2002). *Panarchy: Understanding Transformations in Human and Natural Systems* (1st Edition). Island Press.

Hillman, J. (1972). *The Myth of Analysis: Three Essays in Archetypal Psychology*. Harper & Row.

Jung, C (2010). *Answer to Job*. Princeton University Press.

Jung, C (2014). *The Archetypes and the Unconscious (Collected Works of C.G Jung)* (2nd Edition). Routledge.

Knox, J (2012). *Archetype, Attachment, Analysis: Jungian Psychology and the Emergent Mind*. Routledge.

Lakoff, G & Johnson, M (1980). *Metaphors We Live By*. University of Chicago Press.

Mandelbrot, BB (1982). *The Fractal Geometry of Nature*. WH Freeman and Company.

Meier, CA (ed) (2001). Atom and archetype: The Pauli–Jung letters, 1932–1958. Princeton University Press.

Metcalf, GS (2010). *John Bowlby: Rediscovering a Systems Scientist*. International Society for the Systems Sciences

Miller, J & Page, S (2007). *Complex Adaptive Systems: An Introduction to Computational Models of Social Life*. Princeton University Press.

Pearson, CS (1991). *Awakening the Heroes Within: Twelve Archetypes to Help Us Find Ourselves and Transform Our World*. HarperOne.

Prigogine, I & Stenger, I (1984). *Order Out of Chaos*. New Science Library.

Rahman, T (2025, 26 January). Archetypes and Their Biological Roots. *Psychology Today*.

Stein, M (2006). Individuation. In RK Papadopoulos (ed) *The Handbook of Jungian Psychology: Theory, Practice and Applications*. Routledge.

Stevens, A (2001). *Jung: A Very Short Introduction* (1st Edition). O U P Oxford.

Stevens, A (2006). The Archetypes. In RK Papadopoulos (ed), *The Handbook of Jungian Psychology*. Routledge.

Tinbergen, N (1951). *The Study of Instinct*. Oxford University Press.

2 The Hero's Journey

Joseph Campbell's Hero's Journey

Joseph Campbell noticed similar patterns in mythic stories from all over the world, which he condensed into a generic 'hero's journey'. This distils the common details of all stories and fits them into a holistic story pattern that describes the ebb and flow of life events. His book, *The Hero's Journey: Joseph Campbell on His Life and Work*, takes us from a safe upbringing through an unpredictable and perilous journey during which we must face our dragons to earn the treasure, which is then returned to the people from whom we came. Luke Skywalker, Dorothy, and Harry Potter are all brought up by an uncle and aunt. They all think of themselves as ordinary people, but there is already a hint that there might be some mystery as to why they are not with their parents, and that they might have a special destiny. Frodo is preparing for a birthday party, totally unaware that events are about to change; while Neo in *The Matrix* is an everyday computer hacker.

The Ordinary World

The story begins in a world of innocence. The protagonist is protected until things suddenly change. There is a twist in the story that has sometimes been previously hinted at, which means that life as it has been can no longer continue. Stormtroopers attack the farm where Luke lives, killing his uncle and aunt. There is no farm left. Dorothy is caught up in the tornado. Owls bring secret messages inviting Harry to attend Hogwarts to learn the ways of wizardry. Neo receives a mysterious message on his computer screen telling him to follow a white rabbit. Frodo is invited by Gandalf the wizard to take the ring and use it to save all the hobbits.

The Call to Adventure

The call to adventure is a call to leave behind everything familiar and venture forth into uncertainty. The danger is real and the burgeoning hero often does not feel up to the task. It is hardly surprising that the naïve hero is tempted to deny the call and try to return to their familiar world, if it still exists.

DOI: 10.4324/9781003675266-3

The Refusal of the Call

The call is heard, but for the new hero, it feels daunting. The hero would prefer simply to go back to their previous quiet life. Typically, in fairytales, no return is possible; the only way is forward into the adventure.

Meeting with the Mentor

The mentor who foreshadows what the hero can become appears as a guide. Gandalf reveals himself to Frodo. Obi-Wan Kenobi finds Luke. Dorothy meets Glinda. Harry Potter meets Dumbledore. Neo meets Morpheus and must choose between the red pill and the blue pill. The mentor can only appear when the hero recognises the task ahead. The hero is often given a gift or a power that will later be crucial for overcoming a threat to their pathway forward.

Crossing the Threshold

This is when the prince leaves the castle fair. It is a point of no return. The hero is committed to the journey. Harry Potter goes through the train platform to Hogwarts. Dorothy meets the Munchkins and ventures forth on the Yellow Brick Road. Luke finds himself in Mos Eisley's cantina with many strange and threatening alien creatures from all over the galaxy. Frodo leaves the Shire with the ring, headed for Rivendell.

Tests, Allies, and Enemies

As the hero ventures forth, they meet allies who will help them in their tasks and adversaries who will test them. Dorothy has Toto, the Tin Woodsman, the Scarecrow, and the Cowardly Lion as companions, and the Wicked Witch of the West as her adversary. Luke Skywalker has his group of allies and the evil Empire as his adversary. Frodo had Sam, Peregrin, Merry, and many more as allies, and Saruman and Sauron as his adversaries. Harry Potter has Hermione and Ron as allies and Voldemort as his adversary.

Approaching the Innermost Cave

This is when the hero is now committed to confronting the dragon, which involves moving into the belly of the beast. This is the deep inner journey during which we must face our own darkness. Great courage is needed to keep going, no matter what might be found. Luke and his allies find themselves stuck in the garbage compactor of the Death Star. Jonah finds himself in the belly of a whale; and Dorothy finds herself in the castle of the Wicked Witch of the West. Smaug the dragon provides Frodo with experience of the innermost cave. Stevens (2001) writes of this as a second time in the womb, during which the hero must break free of the mother complex, which gave him birth but now restricts him, so that he can move forward to form a relationship with a woman as an equal partner.

The Ordeal

This is when the hero finally confronts the dragon. It is our personal task to engage with our own dragons. Dorothy must oppose and defeat the Wicked Witch of the West. Luke must face Darth Vader and the Emperor Palpatine in the Death Star. Neo decides to rescue Morpheus, who has sacrificed himself for the others. Frodo must return the ring; and Harry Potter must fight Voldemort.

The Reward

In many stories, the reward for overcoming the adversary is wealth and gold, or the hand of a prince or princess in marriage. This signifies having overcome the adversary and reached a point of completeness. In more complex stories, this is stretched out over several steps. Dorothy is rewarded by being told how she can return to Kansas. Luke finally learns what he needs to defeat the Death Star; and Frodo realises that he can return the ring.

The Road Back

The story is not over just because the adversary has been overcome. In fact, the final challenge still lies ahead. The road back is the return home. From the realm of adventure, the hero must return to everyday life, bringing their gifts with them. Luke and his companions return to the rebel base and are congratulated as heroes. Dorothy finds herself back in Kansas. Neo comes back from the Matrix. Harry Potter is knocked unconscious and finds himself in a hospital bed.

The Resurrection

This is the moment of death – but death leads to a rebirth into something new. For Jesus, this was literal. He died on the cross, descended into hell, and rose again after three days. Dorothy transitions back to ordinary life on the farm in Kansas, but in a new way. Neo is literally shot and killed by Agent Smith, but is brought back to life through the love of Trinity, whose kiss triggers the transformation. Luke's resurrection involves manoeuvring beyond all the defences of the Death Star to fire a missile deep into its core and set off an explosion that destroys it completely. Luke proves himself to be a Jedi knight.

The Return with the Elixir

The final step is the return. The conflict and drama have been resolved – for the time being, anyhow. All parts of the story are resolved. The hero is united with their people and has gifts for everyone. Everyone returns to the Shire, but Frodo and Sam sail off again to start a whole new adventure elsewhere. Dorothy returns to the farm with a newfound respect for the life she has. Neo realises that he is The One and we see hints of what that might mean in his future. We have learned the basic pattern of breathing in and breathing out in life.

Six Archetypes We Live Through

In her book *The Hero Within: Six Archetypes We Live By* (1986), Carol Pearson describes sequences of six archetypes that we live through as we engage in the hero's journey. Each archetype has its own strengths and weaknesses and brings a new challenge that facilitates a more complex, expansive way of seeing the world and opens up more options for how to act.

The journey begins with the innocent, who transitions into the orphan as life reveals itself not to be the perfect dream that the innocent thought it was. The innocent is totally dependent on others to meet their needs, so becoming an orphan is fearful and traumatic. It is tempting for the orphan to turn to addictions to avoid pain. The orphan can tend to seek quick and easy solutions. They may fall for an oversimplified story or someone who promises to reveal the truth. The orphan can unfairly blame others or even become narcissistic, blind to others' pain and demanding that everyone else act in ways that enable them to avoid confronting their own pain. The orphan overcomes despair by transforming into the wanderer, who seeks to resolve the rift in the psyche. By embracing the pain of life, the hero is transformed into something new.

The martyr sacrifices and looks beyond themselves. If not developed well, the martyr sacrifices their core and allows themselves to be controlled by others. They lose their ego attachments by giving to others and sacrificing so that others can gain. Something is put down, but the true martyr picks up more than they have lost, as exemplified by Jesus on the cross.

The wanderer leaves the comfort and security of innocence because they sense that the answers they seek cannot be found in the safe castle. The wanderer ventures forth boldly into an unknown and precarious world. As the prince leaves the castle fair, the dragon stirs within its lair. The shadow is awakened into life and waits for the time when the two must face each other. The wanderer undertakes an inner journey to find themselves. Someone who recently left a relationship embodies the wanderer. They have left behind the security and comfort of the relationship and ventured alone into the future and all that it offers. The wanderer is also the teenager leaving home.

The warrior asserts themselves in the world by acting. However, without the inner looking of the wanderer, the warrior's actions become detached and cause harm. As the warrior acts and interacts, they learn. The martyr needs to change focus from giving to acting and evolving. The warrior has boundaries that they will not allow others to cross. Whereas the warrior tends to use their sword to cut between right and wrong, the magician can embrace the complexity and paradoxes of life.

The magician who follows lives in a different world from the warrior, moving through mysterious realms and unlocking previously unimagined powers to aid in the divine mission. By finding the inherent flow of life, they achieve more than the warrior. The enemy is not so much external as internal – a part of the magician. The magician understands synchronicity. Jung often wrote about how different parts of our world are connected in fractal networks, so there will always be resonances worldwide. If we are alert to their emergence, we can see how our world is held together dynamically and use that resonance to guide behaviour. Following the magician is the return to life and the beginnings of a new cycle with the archetype of the innocent.

Pearson also writes about redefining the hero from the masculine conception that tends to be at the forefront of our minds. She explores a hero who does not need a villain or dragon to conquer. A female warrior is more concerned with maintaining integrity and acknowledging the inner darkness. The martyr gains strength from sacrifice. Pearson notes that men often skip from orphan to warrior, then become stunted and move no more. Women are more attracted to connecting modes, such as the martyr and magician. As with any stage-based model, this is presented as a linear chain for ease of explanation, but in reality it is far from linear. All stages are ever-present, but some move to centre stage when conditions allow. Having the right player centre stage is more important than racing to the final stage.

References

Pearson, C (1986). *The Hero Within: Six Archetypes We Live By.* HarperSanFrancisco.
Stevens, A (2001). *Jung: A Very Short Introduction* (1st Edition). Oxford University Press.

3 The Process of Life

The Tree of Knowledge

Gregg Henriques developed a 'unified theory of knowledge', an important component of which is the Tree of Knowledge (2017, 2022), which describes our journey of evolution from the Big Bang to where we are today and the layers of evolution that we have grown through. This is like a magic key that helps to put things in perspective and unlocks the door to a wealth of understanding of what it is to be human. Henriques describes evolution as a process unfolding over many millions of years, during which we have moved through levels of matter, life, mind, and culture. Matter forms the foundation from which life emerges; life forms the foundation from which the mind emerges; and the mind forms the foundation from which culture emerges. Each new layer is more complex and offers greater opportunities than its predecessor, but it cannot function without its foundation. Let us look more closely at how this evolution has happened.

Matter

Time and space began with the Big Bang. At first, everything was small and dense. It immediately began expanding, releasing enormous amounts of energy. Over time, everything in the universe tends to wind down and wear out. Food rots, mountains erode, animals die. For anything to remain for any length of time, we must create order to counteract the relentless march towards chaos and disorder. We call this wearing down 'entropy'. Entropy in the universe always increases as our world moves towards greater chaos (Bailey, 1990; Odum, 2007).

At the same time as everything began wearing down and moving into chaos, parts of the world became more ordered until they took the form of matter. Atoms were formed with nuclei and electrons that remained stable. Gradually, more and more elements emerged with increasingly complex configurations of protons, neutrons, and electrons. The atoms combined to form molecules, which themselves evolved to become increasingly complex. This was the first realm: the realm of matter.

Eventually, there was a limit on how complex the material world could get. The only way to become more efficient at coping with the entropy was to recombine the molecules in a whole new way. Organic compounds arose. They could form chains of

DOI: 10.4324/9781003675266-4

reactions, meaning that as certain chemicals left the chemical reaction, others came in to replace them, so even though the chemicals came and went, the structure of the molecules was retained. This was the start of life.

Life

Even though life is made from physical matter formed as molecules, it is substantially different from matter. Life can do things that matter cannot. Energy is needed to counteract the wearing-down process through entropy and information is required to organise sustainable structures that hold together. Life requires a flow of matter, energy, and information.

Boundaries and Rules

Instead of the parts all doing what they individually want, they must limit their actions so that the whole system has what it needs to sustain itself. There are rule sets that the parts must obey. This means that all parts of the living system are constrained in how they function. We usually think of constraints as things that hold us back; but here, enabling constraints (Juarrero, 2023) inject order into the chaos and make life possible.

The life-sustaining chemicals must be kept within a bounded environment or they will drift away and degrade. Life needs a boundary (Cabrera & Cabrera, 2015; Juarrero, 2023), such as a membrane, to shield it from harmful external influences and protect what is inside. What is inside the boundary will tend to wear down, just like anything outside the boundary, so there must be a way of bringing matter, energy, and information from the outside in to overcome the internal entropy. Typically, some matter, energy, and information cannot be utilised and must be released back into the environment, creating a flow through the system. Whatever cannot be released remains inside, becoming toxic. Humberto Maturana (Maturana, 2002; Maturana & Verden-Zoller, 2008) describes such living systems as 'autopoietic', based on a Greek word meaning 'self-producing'. Autopoietic systems produce and coordinate what they need to survive from within and do not need anything outside them to control how they work.

Bio-economics

In the same way that we must allocate funds carefully in a business to best utilise the available resources, living systems must allocate their reserves effectively or the system will fall into an energy debt (Feldman Barrett, 2017). Available matter, energy, and information must be transported to where they are needed to power functions such as digestion and boundary maintenance. If anything is not working properly, there must be a repair mechanism. The necessary coordinating infrastructure utilises some of the available free energy.

In addition to internal processes, external functions must be maintained. Living systems must be able to find and acquire suitable matter, energy, and information from the outside world and bring these in through their boundaries. Such resources include food and water. A living system must also be aware of potentially harmful threats in the environment and enact strategies to protect itself so that it can survive. There may be other living systems in the environment that are either food for the system or predators seeking the system as food. These externally oriented tasks are also fuelled by free energy in the system.

All living systems must therefore balance their energy budget, apportioning energy appropriately to manage the entropy both within and outside the system. It is a bit like fighting a war on two fronts: if you send too many soldiers to one front, the other will be unable to defend its boundaries.

We must manage our body energy budget just as we must manage our bank account. We transfer money between accounts to ensure that there are sufficient funds in each account to cover the expected bills. Sometimes we feel stressed and anxious about events in our lives. That feeling of being overwhelmed is like receiving a bill for more money than we have available. We desperately look for ways to economise. Someone else might be willing to take over the debt or perhaps provide a loan. Sometimes no help is available and we must declare bankruptcy. We lose all our savings and must start again from the beginning. When entropy is too great, we become overwhelmed. The toxic effect – whether from bad food, bad emotions, bad thinking patterns, bad social events – affects our social reputation and becomes trapped inside us. Antonio Damasio writes of the same concept, but tends to use the term 'homeostasis' (Damasio, 2022).

Entropy

If I drink too much alcohol, my body will do what it can to expel the matter, energy, and information that it cannot handle. The liver can manage a certain amount of entropy, but it has its limits. What is left remains trapped in the body, slowly poisoning the person until they die.

In the children's game 'Hot Potato', a ball is passed around while music plays. If you are holding the potato when the music stops, you are out. People, therefore, try to pass on the potato as quickly as they can, so that they do not get taken out of the game. The flow of matter, energy, and information is the same. Because entropy involves the flow of matter, energy, and information, people avoid being left holding the excess entropy that they cannot manage.

Choices have consequences. Every time we choose, we reject other options. If we reject certain matter, energy, or information, those rejected choices can often have an impact. If we choose unwisely, we may end up lacking something necessary or we might accept something that proves to be harmful. It is a bit like Isaac Newton's principle that every action has an equal and opposite reaction.

We interact energetically at all levels of our being. We do physical work for others, sometimes giving or exchanging objects. People also transfer emotional, mental, social, and spiritual energy. Interactions between people can result in benefits for both, losses for both, or gains for one at the expense of the other.

Over time, living systems evolved to become increasingly complex, needing more and more energy to sustain life. Eventually, a system becomes so complex that it needs too much energy to maintain itself. The system often falls apart and disintegrates.

Sometimes, it can self-organise in new ways that enable it to continue. Sometimes, a whole new level of complexity emerges at a higher hierarchical level, such as body organs organising as whole-body systems. This higher level can constrain lower levels to cooperate in ways that they had not previously. Whole new layers of functioning emerge. In this way, life has developed layer on layer of hierarchy. This is sometimes referred to as a 'system of systems', where the parts come together to form a system. However, the systems then themselves come together to form a supersystem at a higher level of complexity.

As living multi-celled creatures became more evolved, specialised cells coded and carried information to and from within those creatures. Octopuses have a complex network of nerve cells that helps to coordinate their actions. Each leg of the octopus controls itself independently, but there are cells linking the legs so that they can cooperate coherently as a single creature. Even though its neural system is unlike ours, an octopus is capable of astounding feats of cognition and problem solving. The octopus is pushing at the edge of what is possible within the realm of life.

We have seen how life emerged from matter when matter reached the limits of its ability to reorganise to manage entropy. The realm of life was much more complex and required greater flows of matter, energy, and information. The realm of life similarly met an upper limit with networks of neurons communicating. The pressure to continually evolve and manage entropy led to the emergence of the realm of the mind.

Mind

In microscopic living systems, information can be sent simply by introducing chemicals into the cytoplasm. However, as living systems grew bigger, they became less effective and pathways were needed. Information initially moved through chemical means, but later it was encoded and transmitted by electrical signals using nerve cells. As the message sending became better coordinated, the rudiments of a centralised brain emerged, enabling creatures to become far more adaptable.

And just as they adapted to other creatures in their world, those other creatures adapted to them. If a lion got better at hunting antelopes, the antelopes had to get better at running away or they would get eaten. This creates a feedback cycle where each constantly strives to gain an edge on the other. This is called a 'recursive loop', which allows creatures to adapt more quickly.

Instinct

The first level of minded beings operated from instinct: inbuilt behavioural patterns that did not allow for adaptation, except over many generations. This part of the brain is – albeit controversially – called the 'reptile brain' or 'lizard brain',[1] because reptiles tend only to have a basic survival brain. Their behavioural options are automatic and hardwired in. As we have already seen, each new leap in evolution eventually hits a ceiling beyond which it cannot become more effective without an entirely new emergent level of functioning.

Emotion

The ability to feel emotion requires a far more complex brain with new brain structures. The limbic system evolved, making emotion possible. With emotions, we send ourselves messages about how we feel about an experience and an urge will arise either to approach it because the feeling is pleasant and safe or to move away because it feels unpleasant or unsafe. Henriques (2022) proposes that at the level of minded beings, animals constantly reassess whether an action is worth the investment needed to achieve the goal. He calls this 'behavioural investment theory'.

Some time ago, I looked after someone else's house for a while. A neighbour's cat came around and poked her nose in the open door. She was working out how safe it felt to explore. She would initially sit and watch from a distance, then tentatively move closer and test it out for a while. She was constantly making guesses about the risk to her future if she proceeded into the house.

There are two sides to risk. The first is the danger associated with the action; the second is the severity of the consequences that would result if that danger were to materialise. Since we cannot predict the future, our assessment must be our best estimate.

We actively avoid situations that are likely to happen and would be catastrophic. Other situations would be very unsafe but are unlikely to happen. Dying in an aeroplane crash would be a horrible way to die, but the risk of this happening is low. Many thousands of people cram themselves into metal tubes that hurtle through the air at hundreds of kilometres per hour for the convenience of arriving at a desired destination quickly, despite the risk. Other situations are highly likely, but the impact is low. It looks cold outside and I wonder whether I should wear a jacket. I then weigh up the inconvenience of carrying a jacket around against the likelihood that the weather will turn bad. If I can gather more information, such as from a weather forecast, I can make a more accurate guess. However, at the end of the day, I must still make a guess and decide.

I could see the cat making these guesses as she slunk into the house when she thought we were not looking. The cat used past experience to formulate likely future scenarios for assessing the risk. At any moment, she was ready to turn and race back outside. After several attempts back and forth, she became bolder until she eventually came close enough to smell our hands. We were never able to pick her up.

Even these more primitive aspects of mind can map the world. At the emotional level, the world is divided into safe/pleasant and unsafe/unpleasant, just as a physical map shows safe and unsafe places. We consult our map based on past experience and position ourselves on it, informing us of our safety and guiding us on what to do.

We live for the future, constantly guessing what we should do next. We must continually generate potential future outcomes and assess them for risk, allowing us to choose the best course of action.

Thinking

A major shortcoming of emotions is that they only reveal what we feel at a given moment. Instincts reign over seconds and emotions over minutes, but we become far more effective when we can consider the impact of intended actions over days, weeks, and longer. For this, we need to think. The neocortex evolved to enable the next level of cognitive functioning. We can use logic and common sense to assess any matter at hand. We use our memory of the past to make sense of the present so that we can act now to bring about a preferred future.

As with the other levels, there came a time when minded creatures reached the limit of their evolution and a jump to the next level of adaptation became necessary. Map-making becomes far more accurate and useful when we can reflect on our situation. Thinking allows us to form beliefs and values about the world and how we should act within it. Our beliefs and values inform the decisions that we make, which shape our actions and their consequences. Once we had gained a deeper understanding of our world, we naturally began to explore how we could collaborate to become even more effective. This is the leap to the world of culture.

Culture

People and animals can achieve more when they cooperate, so it makes sense for them to come together to use their cognitive and physical abilities most effectively. Cooperation requires shared understanding. For example, if people speak different languages, they cannot communicate. More than that, minds must be aligned for communication to facilitate cooperation. Culture is the development of shared ways of making sense of our world. Human beings have developed a diverse range of cultures, each tailored to its unique needs and nature. Each culture selects a particular way of seeing the world which, on the one hand, reveals and opens up opportunities, but on the other, conceals unselected possibilities. Differences in culture between groups can be sources of conflict.

There is a tension when any group forms. The group is made up of individuals who have different desires and priorities. Rules are imposed for the good of the group, which may not always align well with the interests of the individuals. There is a tension between autonomy (ie, the ability to do what you want) and connectivity (ie, conforming to the needs of the group to gain the benefits of collaboration). The gains of cooperating must outweigh the losses of individuality.

Several aspects that lay the foundation for the formation of culture are examined below.

Communication

Communication enables the flow of information and is the core of collaboration. Information must be coded in order to be transmitted (Shannon, 1948). When we use language, for example, we use words as a code for ideas. Someone might see a large bird that might be a threat or an opportunity. Maybe it is just cute. They formulate the words, 'Look – there is a bird.' The word 'bird' is just a sound or a shape written on paper. It has nothing in common with the winged creature that it describes. The idea must then be encoded into a word and turned into sounds or encoded into shapes with letters and punctuation. Next, the person must work out the sequence of muscle movements to produce the sounds or letters selected. The signal must then travel to the other person, but it may get lost or degraded along the way. When the signal arrives, it must be decoded in order to be understood.

We might hear the word 'peace', meaning a state of harmony; or we might hear 'piece', such as a slice of pie. Alternatively, the person might be saying 'peas' or 'please' rather indistinctly. The meaning of a word depends on the words around it. Accents and dialects, different tones, and different qualities of voice all impact on the intelligibility of what is said. Communication is by no means just verbal or written. Everything that we do and experience conveys information.

Hierarchy

Life appears in layers. Higher layers structure the organisation of lower layers to make the whole system more cohesive (Ahl & Allen, 1996; Bowles, 2009). Lower levels have an impact on higher layers. Higher layers must be able to constrain lower layers. Hierarchies reduce entropy overall, even though higher layers still create their own entropy. Hierarchy increases inequality because higher levels have greater power to control than lower levels, by controlling the allocation of resources. In human organisations, people selected to undertake higher-layer functions may distort the dynamics for their personal benefit. Membership of the higher layer is established and maintained by agreement or by force.

Hierarchy significantly reduces conflict due to misunderstandings or disorganisation. The rules are designed to prevent behaviours that would erode the effectiveness of the whole system. Paradoxically, hierarchies also create conflict. They often fuel cooperation internally but increase competition and conflict externally. Conflict arises from lower layers challenging higher layers or higher layers imposing their will on lower layers.

Overall, the advantages of hierarchies usually outweigh the disadvantages, so they are generally preferred over non-hierarchical forms. When a new society or community is established or there is a significant change in leadership, there can be a time of chaos until the various roles have been stabilised and the rule set has been determined.

Rule Sets

Rule sets define the shared understanding of those in a society. They define who is a member and who is excluded. Rule sets specify how experiences are categorised and ordered to make sense in a way that is communicable to others and that enables cooperation. Some behaviours are considered acceptable and others unacceptable. DNA has rules as to how atoms and molecules can combine. There are laws of the land designed for our safety and wellbeing. There are unwritten rules, such as how to set a table.

As soon as a rule is established, the possibility of disobeying it emerges because people maintain their individuality. In particular if the rules are unreasonable, a whole cycle of resistance will appear that must be managed. This further depletes the available free energy, making it unavailable for other uses. The system can handle a certain amount of dissent; but if the dissent is too strong, the system becomes chaotic and unable to sustain itself.

There are also challenges from outside the system – especially from other systems that might seek the same resources. These systems will operate on different rule sets and make sense of the world in their own ways.

Justification

Henriques (2024) again has a theory for how cultured creatures operate, which he calls 'justification systems theory'. Once we have language, we can make claims or a declaration about our world. I can say, 'That apple looks good to eat.' This statement can be challenged. Someone might say that it is not good to eat – or even that it is not an apple. I then need to justify my claim or the action that I have chosen. As we form our cognitive mapping of our understanding of the world, we must be able to justify our map to others. Our perceptions, our sense-making, and our actions can all be challenged. Exploring and proving or disproving a justification can be a powerful tool for self-reflection. Henriques writes that our ego is the mental organ of justification, reflecting the image that we have of ourselves. Justification legitimises what we do. Whereas previously, people gained social influence through physical force, those who skilfully justify and convince others can now gain social standing and influence.

Justification systems emerged for groups of people, allowing the world to be justified in a shared way. Culture was established by stating an assumed justified truth explicitly or implicitly among those who hold the culture. Religion and science similarly present justified narratives that define the assumptions held by those who believe in their respective systems.

Social Evolution

Development in the social realm has taken us through layers of social structures, from small hunter-gatherer groups to tribes, to empires, to nations, and to the whole planet (Wilber, 2007). Hunter-gatherers and other early human groups found that they could gain an advantage over other groups by using specialised roles. Individuals focused on what they were individually best suited for. This required more complex social structures, with more rules and controls. Tribes formed. As more tribes formed, conflict grew between them. Alliances and enmities formed over time, resulting in empires ruled by emperors or monarchs.

Sooner or later, of course, the kingdoms clashed. Sub-layers of aristocracy emerged, often from old tribal chiefs who were absorbed into the monarch's court. Increased education and mobility eventually led to the overthrow of traditional monarchies and democracies emerged as the predominant social structure. The advent of democracy has not been smooth and easy. There are still elite people in top positions with access to power that is often abused. Wars are still waged in democracies. Inequality is still plainly evident.

According to Michel Bauwens (2007), there three main parts of society: business, which drives the economy; the commons, which includes most people using shared resources to meet their needs; and the government, which mediates between the others, ensuring that shared rule sets are in place to maintain cohesion throughout the whole system. Bauwens argues that business has taken over the government and the commons.

While all this has been happening, a technological revolution has been underway. We moved from steam to oil and electricity to power our tools and appliances. While technology has provided us with numerous benefits, it has also incurred certain costs. Climate change is a looming threat to our future. After World War II, computers emerged as a significant force. Moore's Law (Brock & Moore, 2006) – which states that the capacity of computer chips doubles every two years – has held sway for the last three decades, vastly increasing our powers of computation for both good and ill. In recent years, we have seen the emergence of artificial intelligence. We have unprecedented access to information that can be used in ways that will revolutionise our capacity as human beings. The jury is out as to whether this will be positive or not.

The Fifth Joint Point

Henriques (2024) suggests that we have now reached the fifth joint point. Each time a new emergent level arises, it does so from a joint point in the previous layer. Somewhere in the cultural layer is a joint point from which a layer that we might call 'spirituality' may emerge. Perhaps it would already be visible if we knew where to look. Henriques believes that we are on the cusp of yet another momentous leap in development, as revolutionary as the shift from life to mind or mind to culture. This time, the shift will be global, which has never happened before. Previously, if life failed in one place, it would arise elsewhere. We might now realise that, given our global interconnectedness, there is nowhere else to turn in the event of a catastrophic collapse.

To be optimistic, the fifth junction could herald a new spiritual awareness that helps us to realign ourselves away from the excesses of the rule of business and lead to a fairer world in which we value taking care of each other and our environment before making money.

The Layers All Interact

As human beings, all the levels co-exist within us, functioning simultaneously. Within the layers are sub-layers, all interacting intensely, harmonising everything so that we live in the world as a single being. Each layer works autonomously with its own rule set and properties, which sometimes clash with the rules of other layers. We must resolve those conflicts within ourselves. An obvious example is the clash between head and heart. Our head inclines us to act one way, thinking things through logically and rationally to arrive at a definite decision. Our hearts can have a very different perspective on the situation, which can drive us in a different direction. It is not that one is right and the other is wrong. The layers all play their part. There are times when we should follow our head and others when we should follow our heart. Wisdom is knowing which layer or layers to listen to in that moment.

The Brain

The layers of evolved human functioning have a loose correspondence to the layers of the human brain.[2] The human body, which includes the brain, is made of matter. The body is the foundation of life and its basic control operates from the instinctual brainstem at the base of the brain, sometimes referred to as the 'survival brain'. It operates on instincts – preformed, automatic behaviours that cannot be modified. The fight/flight/freeze response sits here. The term 'reptile brain' or 'lizard brain' is sometimes used due to the similarities of this part with the brains of reptiles (Feldman Barrett, 2017; MacLean, 1990).[3] Despite the similarities, the reptile brain in humans is also different – especially because it must connect to all the higher brain centres that do not exist in reptiles.

We next have a life layer to our being, centred in the limbic system, which evolved from the brainstem. It did not appear as a whole new layer, but rather as an outgrowth of the previous layer, growing on top. All higher layers are, therefore, directly connected to previous layers. The limbic system is sometimes called the 'mammalian brain' because mammals have a limbic system. The limbic system is linked to emotions and provides us with an immediate sense of how we feel about ourselves and our situation.

The neocortex sits on top of the brainstem and the limbic system. The prefrontal cortex, just behind our eyes, is the centre of our capacity to think and our social skills. These parts are heavily linked to previous levels, so that we can act as one being. The prefrontal cortex is especially active in imagining the future and exhibiting empathy, which distinguishes us from other animal species. Figure 3.1 depicts the broad areas of the brain and their functions.

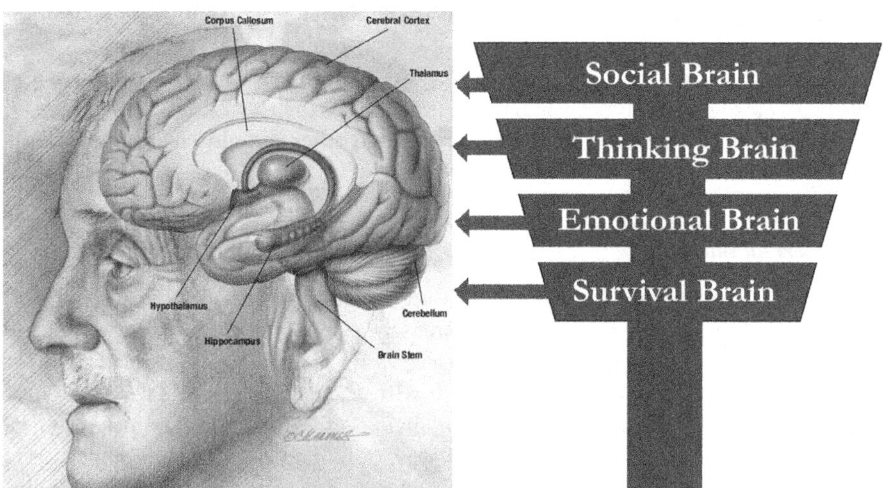

Figure 3.1 A human brain.

This side-on image shows the broad correspondences between parts of the brain and levels of brain function. Source: Wikimedia. Patrick J Lynch. Creative Commons Attribution 2.5 License 2006 Labels added.

The cerebral cortex is divided into two clearly distinguishable parts: the left brain and the right brain. Each side has its own way of operating. They are joined by a group of nerve fibres known as the corpus callosum, which enables them to communicate. Iain McGilchrist (2009, 2021) has examined the left and right sides of the brain extensively. He suggests that the left brain, which controls the right side of the body, tends to be good at concentrating and focusing on one thing at a time. The left side tends to be situated in time and space and is more logical. It categorises everything and pays attention to details. The left side is good at working on things that we already know.

The right brain, by contrast, is more creative. It reaches beyond time and space. It is where art and poetry arise. It has a broad focus, forever on the lookout for whatever might be a risk or an opportunity. It is better at coping with things that we have not come across before. It likes innovation and novelty. This brain works best when we are in a rested state.

There are times when we need to focus on a more logical analysis and others when connecting with our emotions is more important. In general, the more of our brain that is active and functioning, the better we are at responding well to what is happening. Each higher level offers greater complexity for making sense of an event and allows a more nuanced and fit response to be enacted.

The role of the ego is to manage the top-down pressure from the thinking and cultural realms, as well as the upward pressure from instinct and emotion. These must be harmonised so that we can come to one single decision about what to do. The ego conducts an internal dialogue – which we call 'self-talk' – between the culturally shaped narrative self and the embodied emotional self, working out what to decide. It will take the top-down or the bottom-up view and talk about it for a while, gaining more clarity. Then it will swap to the other, gaining further clarity from that side. Having considered two perspectives, we can hopefully formulate a synthesised result. Sometimes the wrong one gets precedence; or we fall into faulty thinking patterns, making our decision-making less effective. Primarily, our self-talk is unconscious, but we can choose to focus and listen to it, and we can choose to change it. Since we can only hold one thought at a time in our self-talk, if we change that one thought, the whole flow changes. We can recognise that we have been too negative and turn to more positive thoughts.

As we know, the levels do not work independently. The limbic system depends on information coming up from the body through the brainstem and input from the prefrontal cortex, adding rationally based information and often inhibitory messages sent to avoid inappropriate social behaviours from leaking out.

We cannot think without access to our emotions. I cannot consider whether I would prefer a burger or a pizza without accessing my emotions. Judgements involve feelings. I must notice what a burger would feel like to eat and then what a pizza would feel like. I must then make a judgement based on the feelings that arise for each option. I might then have a thought – such as, 'The pizza shop is too far away' – which could override the feeling; but the feeling is necessary first.

Each new level can only operate by using the previous levels as a foundation. Thoughts do not magically appear in our cerebral cortex. They arise through all the centres in our brain, from the brainstem to the cerebral cortex. If you think about it, the process of cognition – sensing our world, making sense, and responding – must include our whole being and even the world that we live in.[4] If I want to know whether a nut will fit on a bolt, no amount of thinking will tell me for sure; I must put the nut on the bolt to check whether it fits. Memory is an essential part of sensing, making sense, and responding. We make sense of the present moment by comparing it to the patterns that we have stored in our memory from our past experience. Much of our memory is encoded in the world: I leave a book to take to the library by the door as a reminder. I also write a shopping list, stop at traffic lights, and look at my computer – all of which are part of making sense of my world, so that I know what to do.

Operating the brain is a heavy drain on the body budget. While the brain is only 2% of the body by weight, it uses 20% of the energy that the body has available. The higher the layer in the brain, the more it draws on the body budget. When we move into a state of overwhelm or stress, the call on the body budget exceeds what is available – just as, when our bank balance is in overdraft, we must find a way to economise or the bank will close our account. The easiest way to reduce the drain on the body budget is to shut down the heaviest energy users. That means closing the brain from the top down. The first part of the brain to shut down is the right brain. While this helps with the immediate problem of balancing the budget, the cost is that we lose the capacity given by those brain parts. We lessen or lose the inhibiting functions of the right brain, making it easier for the lower emotional and instinctual brain areas to swamp the higher cerebral cortex. We lose the ability to be creative and think outside the box, which might be just what is needed to solve the problem.

When shutting down the right brain is not enough, the left brain closes down. We lose our capacity to think with any clarity. We lose our social skills. We are not as good at negotiating, empathising, and foreseeing future consequences. Now, whatever emotion is on top will be expressed without the inhibitory effects of the cortex to modulate the behaviour. If the stress is still overwhelming, all we are left with is our basic survival instinct. When we have a disagreement with someone, we try to use our social skills to negotiate and seek mutual solutions. When that fails, we resort to arguing and trying to convince others that we are right. When that too fails, we yell, scream, and cry; when that fails, we fight.

If we trigger our fight/flight response because of a presumed imminent threat, the red brain – the more reactive limbic system and brainstem – tries to shut down all the higher brain processes that might delay acting, which could be fatal. Our early ancestors on the African savannah regularly found their lives under threat, but when was the last time you literally thought that you would die? A wild animal sees its body as its identity. If its body is attacked, its identity is attacked. A human includes their name, nationality, religion, culture, possessions, and so on in their identity. If any of these feelings of threat are triggered, the red brain can activate the fight-or-flight response, so we tend to unnecessarily and unhelpfully trigger our fight-or-flight response when there is no imminent threat.

The dorsolateral part of the prefrontal cortex is designed to rapidly send a message from the cortex to the red brain to inhibit the red brain response from swamping the brain. Essentially, it says, 'STOP AND THINK!' It tries to create a slight delay before the person responds from the emotional and instinctual centres, so that the cerebral cortex can catch up. This usually works well, but sometimes the instinctual reaction overpowers the more considered thought process.

Calming our body state can be very helpful because it helps the right brain to switch on again. Techniques such as breathing can lead the brain to think that the emergency is over, so it stops producing adrenaline, which keeps the body in an alert state. The body then produces chemicals such as endorphins and serotonin, which help to calm us down. Often, we need to move away from the trigger or find a distraction.

You may recall a time when you had a problem that you were concentrating hard on but could not solve. You gave up and walked away. You might have gone for a walk or just stopped for a coffee. That more relaxed state was enough to reactivate the right brain; and suddenly, out of nowhere, you found the answer that had eluded you. It is always helpful to distance ourselves from a problem – to take a break or sleep on it – to allow our whole brain to work on it. It is surprising how often a solution arises.

We may be gaining more control over our red brain over time. For example, the Plantagenet kings of England (1154–1485) were significantly more reactive and impulsive than would be acceptable today. They were capable of extreme violence (Jones, 2014). Partly because of the violence and intrigue that were endemic to the times, anyone who was not as ruthless as their rivals would not survive. Time and again, the kings would order an execution on a whim or in a fit of anger. Ivan the Terrible of Russia killed his own son and heir in a fit of rage and may have caused the death of his son's unborn child.

We now understand how we function as human beings and have many helpful tools in our magic bag to take us on the journey; but there are more tools to prepare before we venture into the world of archetypes.

Notes

1 When we speak of instinct, emotion, thinking, and social skills, we are referring to distinct cognitive processes rather than brain parts. While it is convenient and even useful to link these processes to particular generalised brain areas, it becomes problematic. The brain is so interconnected that the boundaries between brain parts are far from simple and predictable. Much emotional processing occurs in the limbic system, but it relies heavily on connections to the body and the cortex to generate an emotion. A human survival brain must connect to all the higher parts of the brain, making it very different from the instinctual brain of a reptile.

2 The brain is so intensely interconnected that associating a brain area with a function becomes problematic. An example might be the light in a bulb. We might say the light comes from the switch on the wall. I turn the light on and the bulb glows; I turn the switch off and it stops. In reality, a vast network is involved in generating the electricity that powers the bulb. It is tempting to name the trigger as the controller.

3 The brain stem of a human is linked to many higher functions that are not present in the reptile. While many human brain stem functions are similar to those of a reptile, they are not the same.

4 '4e' cognition tells us that cognition is embodied, embedded, enactive, and extended. It requires a body embedded in an environment in which the body acts. Some cognitive tasks, such as memory, extend into the environment, as seen when we use a shopping list. See the works of Evan Thompson (2007), Shane Gallagher (2006), and Andy Clark (2024).

References

Bailey, KD (1990). *Social Entropy Theory*. State University of New York Press.
Bauwens, M (2007). The Peer to Peer Revolution. *Renewal, 15*(4), 25–37.
Brock, DC & Moore, G (2006). *Understanding Moore's Law: Four Decades of Innovation*. Chemical Heritage Foundation.
Cabrera, D & Cabrera, L (2015). *Systems Thinking Made Simple; New Hope for Solving Wicked Problems*. Cabrera Research Lab.
Clark, A (2024). *The Experience Machine: How Our Minds Predict and Shape Reality*. (Herauitgave Edition). Penguin Books.
Damasio, AR (2022). *The Strange Order of Things: Life, Feeling, and the Making of Cultures* (1st Edition). Robinson.
Feldman Barrett, L (2017). *How Emotions are Made: The Secret Life of the Brain*. Pan Books.
Gallagher, S (2006). *How the Body Shapes the Mind*. Clarendon Press.
Henriques, G (2017). *A New Unified Theory of Psychology*. Springer.
Henriques, G (2022). *A New Synthesis for Solving the Problem of Psychology: Addressing the Enlightenment Gap*.
Henriques, G (2024). *UTOK: The Unified Theory of Knowledge*. Sky Meadow Press.
Jones, D (2014). *The Plantagenets: The Warrior Kings and Queens Who Made England*. Viking.
Juarrero, A (2023). *Context Changes Everything: How Constraints Create Coherence*. MIT Press.
MacLean, PD (1990). *The Triune Brain in Evolution: Role in Paleocerebral Functions*. Plenum.
Maturana, H (2002). Autopoiesis, Structural Coupling and Cognition: A History of These and Other Notions in the Biology of Cognition. *Cybernetics and Human Knowing, 9*(3), 5–34.
Maturana, H & Verden-Zoller, G (2008). *The Origin of Humanness in the Biology of Love*. Imprint Academic.
McGilchrist, I (2009). *The Master and his Emissary: The Divided Brain and the Making of the Western World*. Yale University Press.
McGilchrist, I (2021). *The Matter with Things: Our Brains, our Delusions and the Unmaking of the World*. Perspectiva Press.
Shannon, C (1948). A Mathematical Theory of Communication. *The Bell System Technical Journal, 27*(July, October), 379–423, 623–656.
Thompson, E (2007). *Mind in Life*. Belnap Press.
Wilber, K (2007). *Up from Eden: A Transpersonal View of Human Evolution*. Quest Books.

4 Charting the Journey

Introduction

We stand at the threshold between our old secure castle, where we have been safe and protected, and the dangerous, unpredictable real world. Now, it is nearly time to venture boldly forth. Before we leave, we need more tools for our magic bag. The tools will all come together in the dynamics of life model at the end of this chapter.

As we venture into new lands, we will need a map to guide us. Other brave souls have ventured this way before and told of their journeys – all the pitfalls and the struggles that they encountered. Let us explore this guiding map in more detail. The map is a smaller version of the actual terrain that shows the relationships between my location, the places around me, and my destination. An archetype is a particular type of map, mapping my social relations with those around me.

When I arrive in a new land, I look out at the territory before me and recognise some features, such as rivers, mountains, buildings, and more. As I recognise them, I situate myself on the map. I can choose a place on the map that I would like to reach at some time in the future and plot a course between the two points, which provides me with information to help me arrive safely at my destination. I do not just wander at random but have a clear plan. I can identify the most direct route and see where there might be dangers. I know which places to avoid and which will provide me with whatever I need on the journey. Sometimes, maps have errors that I must take into account.

Similarly, when we go to a place that we already know, we have a map in our mind of this place that allows us to get there. It might be an image in our head or a list of directions telling us when to turn. We might turn left after three streets or when we reach the little church, and then take the next right turn. We have a retrievable mental map that enables us to reach our destination. We map much more than physical directions with our minds. Living creatures map themselves, as well as the other people in their lives and the world that they inhabit.

Even a microscopic single-celled paramecium behaves as if it has a plan. It responds to chemical and physical cues in its environment. When conditions become favourable, its membrane remains stable and its cilia drive it forward. When conditions worsen, the cell triggers a brief electrical spike that reverses its ciliary beat, sending it off in another direction. Terrence Deacon describes this as 'entention'. The organism

DOI: 10.4324/9781003675266-5

simply follows built-in constraints with no consciousness at all, but the resulting action appears intentional. The paramecium's map is exceedingly simple, but it has been enough for these organisms to survive for many millions of years. Even flowers have a kind of map, allowing them to track the sun through the day by shifting growth hormones, capturing more energy.

A newborn baby has minimal mapping compared to an adult. They have a fear of falling and a fear of snakes; they are drawn towards pleasant feelings and repelled by unpleasant ones. They already know their mother's voice from inside the womb. A newborn has about 100 billion brain cells, which is about what we will have for the rest of our lives. However, only about 15% of the connections between the brain cells are already set. The way that brain cells connect depends on the environment in which they find themselves. If we find ourselves in a loving, supportive environment, our brain cells will grow in ways that foster openness, confidence, and trust. If we are born into a dysfunctional environment – as so many of us are – we build our brains to cope with a world we perceive as harsh, threatening, and untrustworthy. We create our map as we experience life and tweak it when we find ourselves in error, so that our map evolves and grows with us.

At first, a baby does not even know that they have a body. Everything is just a mix of sounds, smells, and sights that takes a while to make sense of. As the baby interacts with the world, they start to notice patterns (Cosper et al, 2020; Waxman & Leddon, 2011). They notice, for example, that touching their hand, foot, or nose feels different from the cot, the rug, a toy. They slowly build an image of their body as something separate from the environment. This opens a world of duality in which they must live. The baby maps the things that they find pleasurable and the things that they find unpleasurable. When their mother comes into the room and picks them up, they feel safe, warm, and protected. When they are alone, they feel lost, abandoned, and unsafe. Whenever something happens, it becomes increasingly likely that this event will match a pattern from the past that helps the baby to make sense of the present experience and therefore respond more effectively.

As the baby has a limited ability to perceive and understand what is happening around them, they will make errors in their mapping. Children's worlds are often described as magical, where the conclusions about 'what causes what' are inaccurate. If there are errors in a map, we will get lost. We will unknowingly fall into danger and miss promising opportunities that might be right before our eyes.

Our map is formed by past experience because the best predictor of the future is what has happened in the past. We form predictions of likely futures from past patterns. We then analyse each prediction and work out our best response.

As we have seen, evaluating future risk requires assessing the likelihood of an event happening, combined with how bad it would be if it did happen. We must balance the probabilities to determine risk. As soon as we act, we change the situation, so we must constantly re-evaluate the event, formulate new scenarios, and assess the risk to know what to do.

Every time we make a connection that seems to work, we are rewarded with a small surge of dopamine that makes us feel good and motivates us to repeat what worked. George Lakoff believes that these connections are made by neurons physically linking in our brains (Lakoff & Johnson, 1980). Whatever we keep repeating becomes a habit pattern. Our brain physically grows in different ways according to the events of our lives and how we make sense of those experiences. A child brought up in a supportive and loving environment will be wired for trust and confidence. They will be open to new experiences. A child brought up in a less fortunate environment is more likely to learn distrust and suspicion. They will be looking for threats at every turn.

Imagine these two children are in a room when someone they do not know comes in. One will be open and accepting, looking forward to the experience. The other will treat the stranger with suspicion and see them as a threat; they will constantly be on guard for ways in which they might be harmed.

Our brain develops particular skills in sequence, in line with the layers of the mind. At first, the focus is on bodily movements and, a bit later, emotions. Initially, this is basic, such as recognising and copying a smile. Later, tantrums erupt as they cope with emotions. Language and thinking skills are next. Basic skills start early, but critical and logical thinking typically begins to emerge between five and seven years of age. We move on to develop social skills in our teenage years. There is a right time to develop each of these skills. However, this development can be affected if there is a disruption to life during these times. If we learn a second language during the natural time for learning our first language or at least before our teen years, we will find it much easier to learn further languages later on in life.

When growth and learning are disrupted, it is as though a road has been closed and a detour becomes necessary to reach the destination. A traumatic or other disruptive event has disrupted the pattern for developing neural pathways. This does not generally mean that we cannot learn the task, but the neural cells must link less directly. We can still get there in the end, but – like a detour – the route is harder and slower.

Jordan Peterson's *Maps of Meaning* (1999) explores the world of archetypes using the hero's journey and stresses how life arises from the interplay of order and chaos. Peterson describes how we generate maps of meaning, and how it is through these mental maps that we can ascribe meaning to the events of our lives.

Operating the Map

Once we have a map, we can make sense of any new event. I can compare the map to the event. From the map, I recognise relevant patterns from the past and use them to predict likely future outcomes (Friston & Kiebel, 2009; Rosen, 2012). I will see signs in the present moment, such as a hole in the road coming up, that I can assess from past experience to identify the best response.

We can also predict internal events. If I stand up too quickly, there will not be enough blood in my head and I will feel dizzy. To counteract this, as soon as we develop the intention to stand, we increase our heart rate, so that there is more blood in our heads – so by the time I do stand, there is no problem.

As I am walking, I scan the road for anything that might impact my progress. We do this so often that we stop noticing what we are doing. I might spot a blockage across the road. I do not wait until I get to the blockage. I recognise from past experience that I will be unable to pass, so I will search my cognitive map for previous experiences that are sufficiently similar and recall what worked then. I could potentially walk down the next street, find a way around the blockage, or turn around and go home. I will then analyse these scenarios and assess their suitability. They will each have positives and negatives that must be balanced out. If necessary, I will alter my map with the new information.

We are creatures of the future. As soon as we act in the moment, our present situation changes, so future possibilities also change. We create a feedback loop in which our actions change our world and engender new events to be managed. We are constantly in this loop, assessing our present situation by comparing it to our mapping of past events and projecting future scenarios. Once we have analysed the options, we choose our actions and act accordingly.

As we loop through these cycles, we sense, make sense, and respond. These are not three separate events that happen in a sequence. Instead, we are always sensing, always making sense, and always responding. As we make sense of a situation, we may realise that there is important information missing, so we will move our body to sense extra relevant information. Maybe we need to move closer or approach from another angle. Perhaps we need more force, or less, or to focus our senses differently. As we act, we monitor our actions by sensing ourselves both inside our body, to be aware of how we are moving, and outside, to be aware of how our actions are changing the world. If I reach out for a coffee cup, I constantly sense where my mouth and cup are to regulate my movement. Sensing, making sense, and responding constitute one ongoing process.

We rewrite our map by forming new habits. What we repeat often enough becomes a habit. A process such as cleaning our teeth is hard to do the first time, but soon, our brain turns the complex set of coordinated muscle movements into a habit pattern. The brain loves habit patterns because they are very easy on the body budget. Whenever the brain can use a habit pattern, it will. It is a bit like pressing the print button on a computer. You do not need to know anything about how the computer prints a document – just which button to push. When we have repeated something often enough, the brain establishes a habit.

This means that anything we choose to repeat can become a new habit. If we use prayer or affirmations, we are creating new habits. If I change a belief from one of worthlessness and incompetence to one of confidence and competence, my whole being will start working towards making the new habit true.

My map represents how I see myself in the present moment, so my brain will work to create that. If I imagine a better future self and keep telling myself that is who I am, my brain will work to create the future me. There is no guarantee that everything will turn out as you hope, but it is part of growing to become someone better. You may have heard the saying, 'Fake it until you make it.' This principle is used to create a positive future self. When our whole brain is active and all levels are connected and interacting, we are in a focused but relaxed state of mind. What we say and do in that state of mind becomes embedded more quickly and more deeply.

There is an underlying pattern to the universe that is well worth understanding. It reveals the most effective way for energy to flow through a living system.

Fractals

Matter, energy, and information flow through all living systems. Obviously, it will be helpful if the flows are steady and reliable. Any unnecessary disruptions will make the system less effective at managing the entropy within it. Once matter, energy, and information flow into the system, they must be routed as efficiently as possible to where they are needed. Typically, the flow originates from a single source and must be evenly distributed across a network; or it comes from a vast network and must be consolidated into a single source. Think of a tree. The nutrients come from the root system and are drawn up the single trunk and dispersed out evenly, so that all the leaves get the nutrients they need. Other nutrients, such as water and sunlight, can be absorbed by the leaves and transported to wherever they are needed.

What, therefore, is the most efficient way to distribute a resource from a single source to a vast network and vice versa? Imagine a vertical pipe, approximately 12 centimetres in diameter. After 50 centimetres, the pipe divides at the bottom into two 6 centimetre pipes, so that half the water flows down one side and half the other. The two divide like that again and again and again, getting thinner by the same proportion each time. When we pour water down the pipes, we can see that the water flows freely

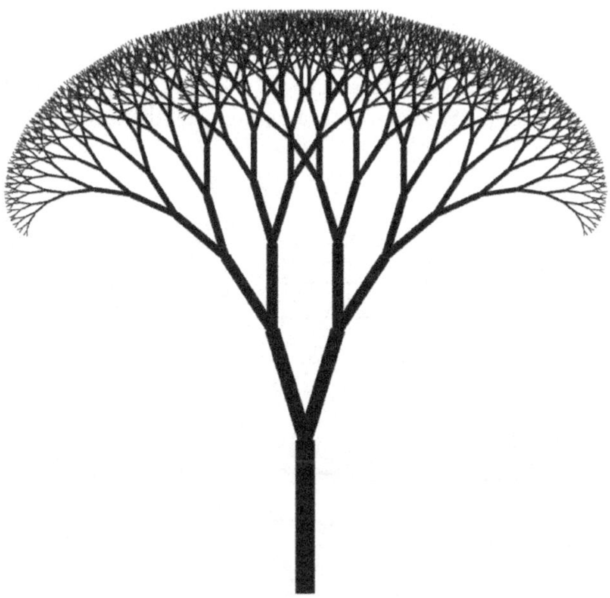

Figure 4.1 A digital fractal version of a tree.

Notice how the tree branches at regular intervals and the branches become progressively thinner. This ensures that sap can travel easily through the whole tree.

Source: Fractal tree, Claudio Rocchini https://commons.wikimedia.org/wiki/File:Fractal_canopy.svg CC Attribution Share Alike 3.0 Unported.

and comes out at the other end in an even stream. If the pipe is divided in any other proportion – say, 8 centimetres and 4 centimetres – we will get blockages and empty pipes. The water coming out of the bottom will flow in stops and starts.

If we then turn the pipes upside down and pour water evenly into all the small pipes, and the proportions are held constant, the water will flow smoothly through the pipes to the one at the bottom. Trees, cauliflowers, our blood systems, computer networks, the nerves in our brain, and so many more things that we see about us every day fit into this fractal pattern to move matter, energy, and information efficiently and effectively from place to place. It is no coincidence that our lungs resemble trees when viewed from above, or that a network of rivers flows down to the sea. This pattern changes by the same proportion at each level and is called a fractal.[1] It is somewhat similar to managing a business, where the flow of income is steady and predictable. You can then forecast your financial needs and plan for times when you know that a big bill is coming.

Fractal structures repeat themselves throughout the environment at different levels. Archetypes appear fractally as recurring patterns within each person within a society that help to coordinate cooperation and understanding within that society.

The Dynamics of Life Model

We are now in a position to introduce my own dynamics of life model (MacGill, 2023), bringing together the threads that we have examined so far. You will note how aspects of the foundational dynamics of living and social systems become encoded into archetypes. The model has three parts. The first (see Figure 4.2), depicts the processes

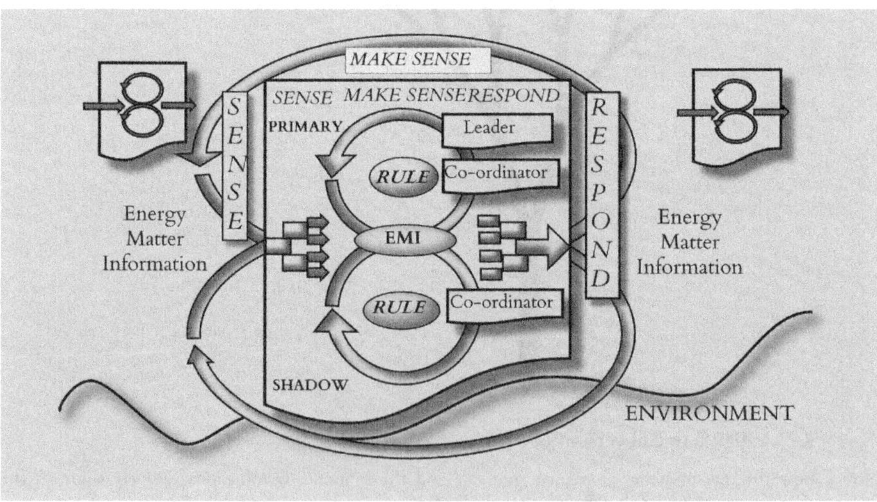

Figure 4.2 The dynamics of life model.

This illustrates how matter, energy, and information flow through any living system.

that take place within any living system to maintain its existence. It is also relevant for subsystems, such as our respiratory or immune systems; and those controlled by living systems, such as an economic or postal system. You will see the inner upper loop, which manages the flow of matter, energy, and information within the body. This includes all body budgeting to ensure that all parts have what they need to do their job. Next, you will notice the upper outer loop, which is the living creature acting in the world and managing itself. It must act to maintain the supplies of matter, energy, and information and avoid any predators or threats that might appear.

The lower inner loop depicts the shadow cycle, which arises from anything that cannot be managed by the top cycle or cannot be expelled back into the environment. The shadow cycle is often toxic to the system's operation and must be managed. The cost of keeping the shadow cycle within manageable limits must be paid for within the body budget. It might manifest as food that cannot be digested or expelled, or an emotion that cannot be consciously managed and is suppressed to remain inside unconsciously, often later reactivated by a trigger event.

A paradox of the shadow cycle is that it often points to what is needed to bring the living system back into alignment. An alcoholic who keeps drinking will generate sickness in their body as a sign of the need to stop drinking. A rival political group may point out how a government's policies harm citizens.

Then there is the lower outside loop, which includes those things in the environment that it must interact with and what has been rejected and expelled back into the environment, which then creates new effects. When we fill a landfill with rubbish, it seems to solve the problem; but sooner or later, a contamination issue must be faced. All our actions in the world have consequences that are carried in the lower outside loop.

Inside the upper loops, there is a model or a map that the living system uses to make sense of the world in which it finds itself. It senses, makes sense of, and responds to what is happening inside its boundaries. A model also operates for the top outside loop and the bottom inside and outside loops.

As we have learned, sensing, making sense, and responding occur by comparing the map to the incoming sensory data. The sensory data must be filtered so that only relevant information is selected; otherwise, the system will be overwhelmed by data (Vervaeke et al, 2009). Of course, we can make mistakes – either by missing relevant information or by acting on irrelevant or incorrect information. The map formed from past experiences to the incoming data is then used to predict likely future outcomes, which are then assessed, leading to a decision and then a response.

Also, within the cycles, there is a storage place for matter, energy, and information. There is often a gap between when a living system can obtain a resource and when that resource will be used. We store matter as body fat that can be turned back into energy when needed. We store information in memory and retrieve it later. As with all things, storage is subject to decay over time. Just as a battery left unused will eventually lose its charge, matter, energy, and information all decline over time, becoming less effective at best and potentially toxic to the living system at worst.

As we have seen with the establishment of a leader, the individual parts within a living or social system find that they are more effective if they cooperate. The more they cooperate, the more they flourish. But there is a cost to cooperating. Coordinating all the parts becomes increasingly expensive for the energy budget. A point is reached where the cost of cooperation becomes greater than the benefits. A group of friends can come together and cooperate very easily. They all know each other and can talk through any problems. One hundred people cannot do this easily. There is just too much work and not enough time. The primary way in which living systems reduce the cost of cooperation is by establishing a leader to make decisions on behalf of the whole. One leader or a small group can easily gather the information needed to make decisions more effectively than the whole group.

As we saw with the establishment of a king, while they solve problems, leadership and hierarchies also create problems. Now, there is inequality. We have the beginnings of a hierarchy. If there is a wise leader, all is well; but sometimes leaders are not as capable as they ought to be, and some will work for their own benefit and to the detriment of the people whom they represent.

Parts within a system may form a new level of hierarchy within the system, or whole living systems may cooperate, creating a hierarchy. If that new level eventually finds that it still cannot manage the entropy that would see the whole system crumble, further layers of hierarchy can be added on top until the entropy is managed. The model shows the hierarchical levels of the coordinator and the leader. Many layers of hierarchy can be added, but each time, inequality increases yet again.

This links to the four layers of Gregg Henriques' Tree of Knowledge to form the second part of the model, which, as we have learned, is linked to the layers of brain functioning. Each layer – the body, emotions, thinking, and social skills – functions as a system in its own right. Sometimes the layers have competing needs that must be resolved. A human being is a system of systems coming together as coherent layers; each has its own identity and individual qualities that coalesce to create a single entity. All four levels are always active in human beings. They interact, and sometimes even compete, so that we sometimes find ourselves flooded by our emotions, which hampers our thinking. As we become stressed, we often shut down our brain from the top down, because the higher levels are more complex and use more bio-economic energy. As we shut them down, we also lose access to those levels. As our social level closes, we lose our ability to have empathy, listen, be open, and look for ways to compromise.

The third part arises from the cyclic patterns in life. Within the dynamics of life model are also the cyclic patterns of life that we have discussed. Living systems undergo cycles that illustrate, for example, how the shadow inevitably emerges as the living system grows, which is akin to the dragon in archetypal terms.

Each layer has its own map with its own priorities and rule set. Each layer has its own reward and punishment systems. The layers are able to negotiate the differences between them in a way that keeps them all functioning and hopefully thriving. They balance each other out, pulling each other back in line when one part strays too far from the allowable limits of the attractors that hold them together.

We can see how societal roles emerge from the dynamics within living entities. The archetype of the king originates from the need to lead through a hierarchy, allowing internal and external processes to be managed effectively. The punishment system becomes the warrior. The stored memory and wisdom become the foundation of the wise person or magician; and the archetype of the lover emerges from the internal monitoring of the system to ensure that it remains within its autopoietic constraints.

Note

1 Fractals were discovered by Benoit Mandelbrot (1982). The Mandelbrot Set is named after him. He coined the word 'fractal' from the Latin word '*fractus*', meaning 'fragmented' or 'broken'.

References

Cosper, SH, Männel, C & Mueller, JL (2020). In the Absence of Visual Input: Electrophysiological Evidence of Infants' Mapping of Labels onto Auditory Objects. *Developmental Cognitive Neuroscience, 45*. https://doi.org/10.1016/J.DCN.2020.100821

Friston, K & Kiebel, S (2009). Predictive Coding under the Free-Energy Principle. *Philosophical Transactions of the Royal Society B: Biological Sciences, 364*(1521), 1211–1221. https://doi.org/10.1098/RSTB.2008.0300

Lakoff, G & Johnson, M (1980). *Metaphors We Live By*. University of Chicago Press.

MacGill, VRD (2023). The Dynamics of Life Model. *Systems Research and Behavioral Sciences, 41*(2), 262–273. https://doi.org/10.1002/sres.2963

Mandelbrot, BB (1982). *The Fractal Geometry of Nature*. W. H. Freeman and Company.

Peterson, JB (1999). *Maps of Meaning: The Architecture of Belief*. Routledge.

Rosen, R (2012). *Anticipatory Systems: Philosophical, Mathematical and Methodological Foundations* (2nd Edition). Springer New York.

Vervaeke, J, Lillicrap, T, & Richards, B (2009). Relevance Realization and the Emerging Framework in Cognitive Science. *Journal on Logic and Computation Advance Access, 72*(1) 79–99.

Waxman, SR & Leddon, EM (2011). Early Word-Learning and Conceptual Development: Everything Had a Name, and Each Name Gave Birth to a New Thought. In U Goswami (ed) *The Wiley-Blackwell Handbook of Childhood Cognitive Development* (2nd Edition), pp 180–208). Wiley-Blackwell.

5 Metaphors

Metaphors Link Our World

In our magic bag, we have another powerful tool to aid us on our journey and help us to make sense of the lands in which we find ourselves. This is the tool of metaphor. Metaphors link as a network to form archetypes. These shared mental constructions shape the whole way in which we see, understand, and map the world that we live in.

Every connection that a baby makes in the world links things together (Lakoff & Johnson, 1980): mother and warmth, a spoon and food, cot and sleep. As we venture into the new world and have adventures, we learn and grow, making new connections, forming the map that we use to navigate the terrain. We connect things that we perceive as having something in common. Every time the baby sees their mother, they notice something different. Her hair might be a little different. Her clothes may change. She might be in a hurry. She might be quiet or loud. Yet the baby recognises that all these different perceptions relate to the same mother. The concept of mother is something new and separate from all the different perceptions, but it enables the baby to make sense of any situation in which the mother is present. Once we have a concept, we can link it to other concepts. In this way, we build image on image to form the basic concepts related to our world. When we link two things, we form a metaphor. We combine things into categories and form patterns in our minds that make sense.

If I had never heard of a woolly mammoth, you might describe it to me as a woolly elephant with longer tusks. Now, something that I had never known before has become known through metaphor. The more we form metaphors, the more predictable the world becomes. We increasingly link patterns to patterns, allowing us to predict situations before they arise and formulate the best response. According to George Lakoff (Lakoff & Johnson, 1980), the essence of metaphor is understanding and experiencing one kind of thing in terms of another. He further suggests that every time we make a metaphor, we are literally joining neurons in our brains. The way that we choose to combine things in our mind shapes our physical brains.

If I have a big bag of buttons, I can combine them in many ways. For example, I could form categories according to colour, size, shape, the number of holes, or whatever. We classify and combine things in the world in terms of categories that suit us and have meaning for us. Inuit tribes have many different words for 'snow', 'ice',

DOI: 10.4324/9781003675266-6

and 'hail', making distinctions that tribes living in warmer areas do not make. We make categories according to the things that are important to us and relevant to our situation.

How we choose these boundaries and what fits within which category can have dramatic consequences. For example, for millennia, certain races have been deemed inferior by others, justifying slavery and all types of discrimination and oppression.

Our world is fractal, so things are linked over and over at different levels. This means that there are parts of our world that suggest they should be linked. Ramachandran et al (2016) experimented with many different cultures around the world. People had to match a cloud-like shape and a spiky shape with the words 'bouba' and 'kiki'. Consistently, the sound 'bouba' is associated with the cloud shape and the word 'kiki' is associated with the spiky shape.

Music links to our emotional states. There is music that feels calm and soothing, and other music that is jarring. Music has a rhythm, just like our body processes. When the rhythm of music resonates with our body rhythms, we feel calm. If music is loud, it tends to link to intense emotions. If it changes suddenly, we are surprised. Music can be used to build motivation and energy. It is inherently connected to our emotional states. We can thus use music to change our emotions, calm ourselves down, or energise ourselves.

Our language is heavily based on metaphors, as concepts are built upon other concepts over time. We talk of 'grappling' with a problem as though it were something that we can hold and push and pull. We speak of a meeting that went smoothly as 'plain sailing'.

Many things in our world seem to suggest links. Good weather signals good times, while stormy weather indicates troublesome relationships. In all languages that I am aware of, time and distance are linked. We can reach a goal or destination in time or in space. Something that is a long way off takes a long time to reach. We encounter obstacles along the way that delay our journey in both time and space. We often link the metaphor of a journey from one place to another to a project or a relationship over time. We have our ups and downs along the way. We talk of the path to success and being on the final lap. We speak of an easy path or being lost in a fog.

Earlier forms of life had to develop maps that distinguished between what was safe and what was unsafe so that they knew what to do whenever they encountered something. If it was safe, it would be approached and valued. If it was unsafe, they would move away from it. A light-filled environment is more likely to be perceived as safe, so light is preferred over darkness. What is visible is easier to notice, so both threats and opportunities are more easily recognised in the light. Up is preferred to down, as in the military rule to 'take the high ground'. You are in a better place to protect yourself if your enemy is below you rather than above you. The higher up we are, the wider the view to identify resources or predators. The front is preferred to the back because our senses have evolved to the front, so that we can focus our attention on what is relevant. If an enemy is at our back, we are much more vulnerable. Warm is preferred to cold because it indicates health and safety.

Open is generally preferred to closed or hidden because it is known and predictable, although sometimes we feel more protected if we are hidden away. We also developed a general preference for right over left. Ninety per cent of people are right-handed. Approximately 25% of handedness is determined by genetics, while the remaining 75% has social causes. If a predator were in front of us, we would not want to waste time deciding which limb to use to defend ourselves. It makes sense to automatically prefer one over the other. It could be because our left brain, which controls the right side of our body, is better at focused tasks that we have a preference for the right-hand side; or maybe this preference just arose by accident.

Thus, very early on, we developed metaphors linking light, up, front, warm, open, and right to feeling safe; and dark, down, back, cold, hidden, and left to feeling unsafe. When we evolved to form minds, rather than devising a whole new set of metaphors, we copied and adapted those developed for navigating the physical terrain to our realm of mind. What was safe and unsafe now became linked to good and bad.

Light became seen as good. If we shed light on something, it becomes visible. If we shed light on a problem, it becomes understood. To lighten up is a pleasant sensation. Darkness is often perceived as dangerous and ominous. A bright, sunny day is often associated with good times when all is well; but stormy, dark weather can be dangerous and uncomfortable. Black is the colour of the devil. Red also has evil connotations because of its connection to blood, which, when spilled, portends injury, loss, and even death. To be caught red-handed is to be caught with blood on your hands. The colour red is often used to catch our attention, such as in a red traffic light, or to indicate an emergency.

We hold dark secrets. They are hidden away from view – a concealed fact, just like an object under cover. If someone has a cold nature, they are not welcoming and friendly; whereas a warm-hearted person is someone whom we are generally attracted to. To progress is to move both forward and upward. We are closer to our goal. If a business does well, we say that things are looking up. We graph the progress and the line heads up and across the page.

Metaphors link to a whole way of seeing the world. We often use military metaphors, especially in the business world. We aim for targets and plan an advertising campaign. We talk of an uphill battle, the war on drugs, biting the bullet, closing ranks and dodging a bullet. We hold fire and lie low. Without realising it, we often shape how we see the world in terms of a battle. How different would it be if our metaphors were more wholesome and life-supporting?

When we have an interlaced matrix of metaphors, it creates an internally consistent way of seeing the world that becomes the basis of our mental map. We can call this our 'worldview'. It is internally consistent among those within the culture for which it is true. In this way, metaphors can come together as an archetype. Other groups and cultures have their own maps and unique archetypal forms. There is always a distortion between our map and the world that we live in.

We discussed how the concept of mother arises for a baby. This happens for all the other people in the baby's world. They formulate generic concepts for men, children, older people, family members, strangers, and so forth. They come to understand the social roles that people play in their society. These become archetypes that live in the psyche of each individual, shaped by the particular culture in which that person is immersed. These archetypes allow us to categorise people as we encounter them and, based on past experience, to make reasonable guesses about each person and how to respond to them. Of course, if our experience of social roles is distorted, our perception of the archetype will be distorted to match.

In traditional societies, competing for survival against rival tribes, even small advantages could mean the loss of fitness in their niche, which could spell the difference between life and death. A tribe that best utilised its advantages – such as physical strength, leadership, or nurturing – would gain preferred access to the available resources. Differentiation into separate roles builds fitness for the society as the attributes are more effectively utilised.

References

Karthikeyan, S., Rammairone, B., & Ramachandra, V. (2016). The Bouba–Kiki phenomenon tested via schematic drawings of facial expressions: Further validation of the internal simulation hypothesis. *i-Perception*, 7(1), 1–6.

Kauffman, SA (1995). *At Home in the Universe: The Search for the Laws of Self Organisation and Complexity*. Oxford University Press Inc.

Lakoff, G & Johnson, M (1980). *Metaphors We Live By*. University of Chicago Press.

6 Sex and Gender in Archetypes

Introduction

As we venture forth on our journey, we hear stories from the past about the people who have walked the path before us. They once trod where we will tread. Some of their stories are indeed heroic and give us hope to move forward and create better futures. However, there are also stories of tragedy and loss, as well as accounts of considerable violence and evil. There is much to learn from them. There is value in looking back to where we have come from to understand how our world came to be and perhaps gain insight into where our future journeys may take us.

As we place ourselves on our map, we recognise that this weather-beaten map, drawn long ago by our forebears, contains errors. The terrain has changed since those bold early travellers drew their charts, and they did not always see things as they are. We are left feeling lost and need to redraw the maps to fit the terrain that we observe today.

Our archetypes evolved with us as we moved from the savannah into towns and into massive cities of many millions of people. Each culture found its own expression of the core archetype that fitted the geography, technology, and social structures around it. Archetypes thus shaped the culture and the culture, in turn, shaped the archetypes. Any errors in the mapping of a society's worldview become embedded in the archetypes.

We are creatures of habit and do not like change because it is bioenergetically expensive and risky. The need for change must generally outweigh the cost and risk, making us wary of change. Often, we must hit rock bottom before we finally make the necessary change. An unfortunate consequence of this is that archetypes are slow to adapt and slip out of step with their society. Archetypes continually recreate and reinforce old, maladaptive patterns, thereby supporting the status quo, even when it is harmful to the people within that society.

Sex and Gender

Sex and gender are deeply embedded in life. Sex and gender influence life at every layer of our being. Our sex relates to the physical body that we are born with; while gender relates to the social constructions that we have developed, particularly shaping identity and what behaviours are appropriate and expected.

DOI: 10.4324/9781003675266-7

As we evolved over millennia, our sexuality evolved in step. Just as some of our brain functions that evolved perfectly for their time later became problematic as our world changed, aspects of our sex and gender have become problematic.

Sex and gender are evident in all the layers of evolution that we have explored. They express themselves differently at the levels of life, mind, and culture. Our DNA and the nature of our physical body shape us at the cellular level. This is the foundational layer that is the least amenable to change. However, modern-day technology has even enabled us to substantially change our physical bodies through hormone therapies and surgery.

Warren Farrell (1993) describes men as the disposable sex. If a large proportion of men in a society were to die, that society could still reproduce itself into the next generation. Women bear the coming generation, so having them undertake dangerous tasks such as warfare is a poor survival strategy. The greater physical strength of males makes a significant difference in traditional societies. It makes sense for men to undertake more physically strenuous tasks. Men may not be so disposable if women become too vulnerable. The traditional values of seeing men as providers and protectors, and women as nurturers, arose because these were effective survival techniques in traditional societies and became embedded in social structures, forming archetypes.

For men to be willing to risk danger and death requires a dampening of emotions. A man must do what is needed for survival in the moment, irrespective of the emotional cost. The world for men today is not usually life-threatening, but this emotional detachment often remains notwithstanding. Men focus on the skills they need, such as being rational, making good decisions under pressure, taking risks, and organising into effective hierarchies to coordinate protective tasks. Rivalry and jealousy arise as the biological constraints are lived out in social relationships.

At a basic biological level, and particularly in more traditional societies, women are more vulnerable than men, especially since only they can have children. If their man cannot protect and provide for them, life becomes precarious. Again, from a biological perspective, men tend to be attracted to youthful physical beauty, as it implies good childbearing capabilities. Women, on the other hand, tend to be attracted to status and wealth, which suggest that their survival needs will be met. Men and women who are highly sought as partners tend to be attracted to each other, meaning that those who are less well-endowed are also attracted to each other.

These biological and psychological ideas form the foundation on which we build our social and cultural agreements. They become codified into social roles and into archetypes, which express the good and bad qualities of men and women. Biological tendencies, therefore, become solidified through social structures and become part of a person's identity. The idea of 'women and children first' is deeply written into modern culture. The more women are seen as the vulnerable sex, the more they become trapped in subservient social roles. As technology improves, we have more options for regulating our societies to be more equal and fair.

Sex and gender impact how we express our emotions and what emotions predominate (Fischer et al, 2004). It is the same with our belief systems. There are clear gender preferences, with significant overlap in how we see ourselves and the world we live in.

Gender differences are evident at the cultural level, where social conventions are established. Gender is far more amenable to change than sex. Sex still places constraints on what can be societally adopted. Social conventions have changed immensely over the centuries to meet changing social circumstances. Equality of the sexes is generally held to be the goal of modern societies in the Western world. We still struggle to resolve how we can act with equality when there are clear differences between the sexes and genders. Men and women can never be equal in the sense of being the same. We must find expressions of equality that embrace our differences. While the similarities tend to be greater than the differences, there are still clear differences.

When social groups compete for resources, minor differences are accentuated. Social roles must be formulated that optimise strengths and neutralise weaknesses. Enacting male and female roles helps to strengthen the fitness of a society compared to its rivals. Any slight advantage in how social roles are enacted could mean the difference between the continued existence of a society and its demise. This was particularly true before technology provided ways to even out the impact of these differences.

Differences between Men and Women

It is clearly an error to deny biology and claim that everything is cultural and therefore totally malleable. Traditionally, men have been seen as providers and protectors, while women have been viewed as nurturers. There are always significant exceptions to generalisations about the nature of men and women, but there are general trends. Men are seen as fixers and tend to be more interested in mechanical objects. Women tend to be more interested in the home, relationships, and personal appearance. Much of this arises from cultural expectations, but there is also a biological component. Experiments with Barbary monkeys (de Waal, 2022) revealed a clear preference for males to play with trucks and guns, and females to play with dolls. If a male plays with a doll, it usually ends up ripped into pieces. This demonstrates that there are deeply embedded innate influences that are not socially constructed.

Generally, men have greater upper-body strength than women. Men are generally expected to undertake the heavier and more hazardous tasks and to be prepared to make the ultimate sacrifice for their country. We send bakers, accountants, and teachers to war as soldiers, and their deaths become acceptable. Higher levels of testosterone tend to make men more aggressive and less agreeable. Women have wider hips to facilitate childbirth, which can impact their mobility. It was long thought that male and female brains were substantially different, but more recent evidence does not back this up (Ryali et al, 2024).

Our anatomy and physiology influence social roles, and over time, our social roles can impact on our anatomy and physiology. The greater strength of men could have led to them being assigned hunting and fighting tasks, while women were more tied to childcare. This might suggest that men would have needed to develop a more focused mind to target prey or enemies, while women would have needed a more multitasking mind to manage the wide range of threats to themselves or those they care for – although the evidence on this is mixed (Mantyla, 2013; Stoet et al, 2013).

Men are enculturated to be unemotional. In an emergency, a man is often expected to remain stoical and strong for everyone else, but there is a cost to this. Suppressed emotion eats away at the core of our being, so men generally have less access to their emotional lives and are susceptible to depression (Real, 1998).

We have seen that the lowest layer that we can use to resolve difference is the physical, which means fighting. Given that men, in general, have a significant physical advantage, women often have a deep-seated sense of vulnerability. In a situation such as walking home at 2:00 am with poor street lighting, a man is not usually concerned for his safety, whereas a woman will feel unsafe. Women know that if a situation becomes physically violent, they will usually end up worse off. This has significant implications for psychological wellbeing.

Women have been portrayed as the weaker sex, implying an inferiority. The disparity between physical capabilities has been generalised to their whole being. They are less likely to use physical violence and will generally employ other means to defend themselves and attack others. Just as misused physical superiority can lead to violence, misused female aggression can tend more towards manipulation (Debowska et al, 2015). Social factors may also be involved. Repeated unmet requests by women, especially for something that they cannot achieve without help, are often experienced by men as nagging.

Some people would suggest that while women generally like to maintain a sense of equality in a group and focus on relationships, men are more likely to find their place in a hierarchical pecking order and are happy to submit to someone higher in rank (Schmidt Mast, 2004). Again, this is contested (Kanter, 1976). Hierarchies speed up decision-making. Those higher up the hierarchy need all the skills and resources available to make the best decisions. Not everyone needs to know the background information that led to those decisions, as long as the leader can be trusted to make good decisions on behalf of the whole or has a wise support base. That is not always the case, and the results of an incompetent or manipulative chief can be catastrophic. A flatter, more even group structure creates a fairer group that encourages collaboration and group coherence, but the decision-making process is slower and more cumbersome.

The most critical difference between hierarchies and flatter social groups is that hierarchies can scale up more effectively. A hierarchy adds more layers, with each layer responsible to the one above. A flatter structure cannot be maintained as easily as more and more people are added. There is not enough time for the necessary relationship-building and social interactions.

Hierarchies have their own conflicts. They create inequality, and people often feel that those higher up do not understand or care for them. There is always someone to challenge the existing structure and attempt to wrest control from those in power.

Group selection, like all forms of natural selection, can be very brutal. There are clear winners and losers. Whatever society is more effective in a given environment gains access to the resources, and the less fit lose those resources, making them even less able to challenge the predominant group.

'For whoever has, to him more will be given, and he will have abundance; but whoever does not have, even what he has will be taken away from him [Matthew 13:12]' (Nelson, 2018). Hierarchies are generally able to organise more quickly and effectively, and therefore to outmanoeuvre flatter structures. Over time, this has led to male-dominated hierarchies gaining control of social structures.

Once men secured prominence in positions of power, they controlled the social position of women. Men could impose their chosen rules to maintain their positions of power. Men actively established social structures that entrenched their positions of power, determining the social status of women, other races, nonbinary genders, and more (Eisler, 1988). One of the main control tools was to impose the acceptable social narratives, heavily shaped by the archetypes that arose from those narratives and that reinforced the existing power structures.

Since archetypes and myths are so entangled in the rule sets of any society, gaining control of the myths and metaphors became a powerful weapon in establishing a patriarchal-based society. Rather than annihilating conquered societies, the more usual approach was to subsume them into the new culture. The captured women often became slaves or wives, who subsequently brought up the children of the dominant culture, meaning that the stories of the old culture remained alive. Typically, patriarchal myths emerged in which the previous goddess was killed or became a consort of the male god. Athena is not born through a maternal lineage but is instead produced from the head of Zeus – a narrative that symbolically transfers generative power from the female body to the male intellect. This shift reframes feminine authority as something authorised and contained by male sovereignty, rather than emerging from an autonomous goddess tradition.

Gender and Societal Roles

An exploration of the evolution of social organisation over the millennia provides insight into the impact of gender-based social roles and the archetypes that evolved. The earliest human societies were more egalitarian. They generally lived in small, extended family-based communities of around 30 people (Manning, 2023; Wrangham, 2019). There was no point in having more possessions than could reasonably be carried on one's back and no need to claim a particular area of land. They moved from site to site as food sources became available. Archaeological sites confirm the equality of group members (Politopoulos et al, 2024). If conflict arose, there was plenty of land for any group to move on to. There were no weapons to fight with.

The stories and myths of this earlier age reflect the people's nature and lifestyle. Often, matriarchal stories and images of goddesses predominated. They were shamanistic and focused on ancestor worship.

For a long time, if a dispute arose within a tribe, a portion of that tribe would relocate and establish a new tribal unit in a different location. Eventually, of course, populations increased so that – in some places at least – land became contested. A place that afforded easy access to vital resources became a prized location. There had to be some way to decide who had a rightful claim over a certain area of land. Agricultural societies became more productive. They could grow and store food, so the supply was more reliable, even if the quality of the diet decreased (Bowles, 2009). For a long time, both ways of life existed side by side. Eventually, agricultural societies proved to be fitter.

It became worthwhile to have possessions and tools. Art and craftwork emerged. Distinctive art and craft styles helped to distinguish groups and generate group identity. Permanent buildings were built for storing food and living in, providing better protection from natural events such as storms. Tools improved productivity.

The ancient city of Çatal Höyük in Turkey, founded around 7500 BC, is an interesting example of a city that does not appear to have been organised in a top-down hierarchy (Hodder, 2006). It had a population of 5,000–7,000 inhabitants with no public buildings, only private dwellings. The art – such as murals and carvings of deities and rituals for the dead – suggests a complex social structure, but there are no signs of weapons or conspicuous wealth. Archaeological evidence suggests a partnership society rather than a matriarchal one.

There is a smaller and older settlement at Göbekli Tepe in Turkey, dating back to at least 9500 BC, also without weapons or signs of hierarchy (Schmidt, 2010). Göbekli Tepe's monumental architecture consists of more than 200 T-shaped limestone pillars arranged in circular and oval enclosures. Some pillars reach five metres in height and weigh several tonnes, indicating that large, coordinated groups were required to carve and position them. Göbekli Tepe was probably not inhabited permanently but may have been a religious site that local hunter-gatherers visited for ceremonies. These sites serve as a reminder that alternative ways of organising, which do not rely on dominance and control, might be possible and offer some hope as to what our future could be. In general, however, the trend all around the world has tended to be male-dominated.

In their book *The Dawn of Everything* (2021), Graeber and Wengrow correctly highlight the extraordinary number of exceptions in larger-scale non-hierarchical societies. They further note that hunter-gatherer societies tended to come together regularly in much larger groupings, such as for potlatch ceremonies, for shorter periods of time and were often more structured in this epoch. Over time, agricultural societies overtook hunter-gatherer societies, so the core social structures had to adapt.

A claim to land by a group was valuable and had to be defended. There was now value in forcefully seizing the land occupied by someone else, taking their stored food, possessions, and tools. This created a need for warriors to defend the territory. Weapons became necessary. Weapons that were initially created for defensive purposes could also be used for offensive purposes, to appropriate the resources of another area.

The art of warfare developed. Weapons and military strategies and tactics, fortifications, and the like became integrated into everyday life. The male advantage in terms of physical strength and the tendency to excel under hierarchical structures led to a male-dominated warrior ethos. Any tribe that could not defend itself against warlike neighbours would perish.

Once possessions were gathered under patriarchal ownership, women became commodities just like livestock, with a monetary value. If land and possessions were to be handed down to a son, it became necessary to ensure that the son was a rightful heir, so rules on chastity were established.

Another consequence of the conquest of tribes was the institution of slavery. The conquered people could be used for menial and heavy tasks. The use of slaves led to a significant increase in productivity and widened the gene pool. Any tribe that did not use slaves would lose fitness compared to rival tribes with slaves and would lose access to vital resources.

These emerging hierarchies and power asymmetries created the cultural and psychological conditions in which recurring symbolic patterns could stabilise, eventually forming the archetypes that exert such a profound unconscious influence on human behaviour. As patriarchal structures came to prominence, myths around the world arose in which the previous goddess was either defeated or married, so that a male god took precedence (Campbell, 1991). The mythology of a society reflects both its creative ideals and its structural inequalities.

Marduk, the Babylonian male god, defeated Tiamat, the earth mother, who is sometimes represented as a serpent or dragon. The world was fashioned out of her corpse. In India, Indra killed Vritra, the mother goddess, and her son, who was also described as a serpent and a demon. Indra then became supreme in the heavens. In Ireland, St Patrick fought with the snake goddess Corra. He was devoured by the snake, but fought his way out and turned her into stone. The Hebrew testament of the Bible and the story of Adam and Eve show all the signs of a patriarchal retelling of an older, more equal story.

As villages became cities within empires, they required increasingly sophisticated organisational structures. Cities necessitated the reliable storage of large amounts of information for trade, taxes, agreements, and other purposes. Writing provided a consistent, accurate way of keeping records over time. Legal codes enshrined in the rule sets became divinely established, as in the Ten Commandments and the Code of Hammurabi. Laws were first written in stone to maintain enough order for the social processes to evolve. Any tribes or societies that did not update their technology were increasingly left behind (Wilber, 2007a).

The larger the society, the more layers of hierarchy that were needed to manage entropy. Leaders had to learn the skills of influencing others to maintain the rule set. Each new layer increased effectiveness but also increased inequality and the potential for entropy to arise from the conflict between layers.

Rule sets form the foundation of the limits on behaviour and actions, holding the group together. Roles were needed to ensure compliance with the rule sets. Roles were needed to maintain and extend tribal knowledge and plan for the future. Roles were also needed to care for more vulnerable members, establishing a maintenance and repair mechanism for the society.

Over time, whether genetically or socially motivated, certain roles tended to be associated with specific genders. The stronger the gender differentiation in a society, the more pronounced its manifestation in the female archetypes.

Archetypes formed during the foundations of our civilisations reflect the values and qualities of those times, but they remain in our present-day psyche. The world that we live in today is immeasurably different. City life bears virtually no resemblance to the environments in which our early ancestors lived. On the savannah, we moved constantly: running, jumping, chasing, carrying loads, swimming, and so much more. We do not need to move our bodies as our forebears did to undertake our daily tasks, but we still need to exercise – perhaps by going to a gym. If we do not, our bodies – still optimised for the savannah – will become obese and unhealthy.

In the same way that our bodies' archaic needs must be met, the archetypes that evolved on the savannah cannot be ignored. They still impact on modern-day life. There is a mismatch between the cognitive mapping that we inherited from our ancestors and the mapping of our modern world.

We discriminate against whatever can be easily distinguished. Gender and skin colour are plainly visible. People with red hair may face discrimination. The first wave of feminism arose out of the wealthy middle class who could afford servants in the late 19th century, so some women were freed to consider what more they could be. After World War II, women had to undertake the jobs of men who had left to fight and proved themselves more than capable. Contraception gave women a choice over having children, while household appliances such as refrigerators and vacuum cleaners freed up time for all women (Freedman, 2002).

The physical advantage that men once had is largely gone now. Machines or computers do most of the heavy or difficult work. Opportunities emerged for women to pursue careers. There is still discrimination as we struggle to come to terms with how to enact equality. There have been unintended consequences of needing two incomes for families to survive financially, including the impact on childcare and the phenomenon of empty suburbs as both partners leave to work.

Attitudes to race have similarly changed over time. While many steps have been taken towards equality, the impacts of colonialism remain firmly entrenched and we are far from living without racism.

There has also often been a preference for the firstborn throughout history, including in European culture and in the New Zealand Māori culture (Mead, 2016). The firstborn ('*Tuakana*' in Māori) takes precedence over those born later and will speak on behalf of the family. If you think of earlier times when people had larger families, the fortune that a man amassed over his lifetime would be wasted if each child just received an equal portion. None of the children had a sufficiently strong resource base to succeed. If one child, the firstborn male, gained a significantly greater share, it was more likely that the family dynasty would survive. This arrangement provided the entire family with a way to maximise opportunities. There was an understanding that the firstborn had an obligation to their younger siblings, and hopefully, their greater opportunities meant that all could do better than they otherwise would have.

We like to think that we make changes towards a more equitable society because we realise that what we did previously was wrong. However, human beings have an immense capacity to remain blind to suffering when the maintenance of a certain lifestyle is at stake. The changes had more to do with the search for more efficient ways of getting work done (Mathias, 2001). Slaves had to be fed and controlled. They always tried to escape. When machinery became available that could do most of the tasks that slaves had previously undertaken, we were free to see slavery for what it was. It was the same for women's rights – as it is now for climate change. We know what is needed to mitigate climate change, but until we have a viable alternative, we not only continue using fossil fuels but also are using them faster in case another nation takes advantage of our sacrifices for the good of all humanity.

Over the last few hundred years, and particularly the last century, we have seen deeply entrenched views on slavery, sexism, racism, and gender more radically challenged. We have come to realise how people have been dominated and persecuted. Generation on generation has suffered and been denied justice. Minorities have rightly stood up and contested the established society, which perpetuates harm.

The clear hegemony of the Catholic Church was challenged by Martin Luther and the Protestant religions (Melloni, 2017). People now saw a pathway to God other than through the Catholic Church; but the Age of Enlightenment revealed a world that could exist without God. Nietzsche claimed controversially in the 1880s that God is dead (Nietzsche, 1964), and that we killed God. He argued that the Age of Enlightenment had introduced a materialistic perspective on the world, undermining the previous worldview, which had remained virtually unchallenged for hundreds if not thousands of years. Dostoyevsky wrote in his novel *The Brothers Karamazov* (2002) that if God is dead, anything is permissible.

The death of God pronounced by Nietzsche heralded a descent into what John Vervaeke calls 'the meaning crisis' (2019). There is now no absolute universal truth, but only each person's own truth, with no truth being more valid than any other. As a global society, we have lost our uniting story. Postmodern philosophies that arose in the aftermath of Nietzsche's proclamation certainly have their value in highlighting the iniquities of past worldviews, but they have also left us drifting aimlessly like an unanchored boat on an endless ocean (Gemes, 2001).

Life today moves at a pace that the archetypes cannot keep up with. Issues of race and gender, in particular, are highly controversial. Whenever we pare down stories to their bare bones and hold just the essence, there is an inevitable simplification. Good and evil are generally portrayed in fairytales in very binary ways. The goodie wears a white hat and the baddie wears a black hat. If we are truly prepared to step back and see the bigger picture, the murky grey area between good and evil is substantial. We are all a mix of both and often delude ourselves about our goodness.

Gender is similarly generally portrayed in fairytales as male or female (Shaheen et al, 2019). There is no substantial archetypal development of alternative genders. Today, movies are the driving force behind new mythological forms. The moving image is generally more appealing than the written or spoken word. In time, archetypes will change as more and more aspects of our psychology are brought to light. We are certainly seeing female heroines play a more prominent role in movies today – often in mythologically based stories such as *Star Wars*, *The Lord of the Rings, Harry Potter*, and *The Matrix*. *Star Trek* pioneered other genders and races as the crew of the Starship Enterprise.

The archetypes that we choose to bring to life will determine the direction of our future. The metaphors that we use are also very powerful. George Lakoff (2014) demonstrated how we tend to use militaristic metaphors in the business world and in politics. We talk about 'gaining the higher ground', 'winning the battle', a 'political campaign', 'sales targets', and so much more. We could have chosen to focus on the positive side of the mutual exchange of goods for trade rather than defeating an opponent. Feminists have long recognised the value of challenging patriarchal terms such as 'chairman', 'salesman', 'policeman', and 'fireman'. The more these words are used, the more they reinforce unhealthy social norms. In many ways, we have changed the battlefield from a geographical space to a field of communication, where a battle is won by influencing minds. The language that we use is extremely powerful and the movies that we make have a major influence on how we conceive our future.

As much as we can learn from the myths and fairytales that we choose to create, our traditional stories speak directly to deep unconscious motivations within our being. While we can change our archetypes over time, those that persist remain as powerful influencers of our individual and collective behaviour, whether we like it or not. We must, therefore, be cautious in what we take from archetypes and how we use them, because if we do not use them wisely, we perpetrate the very sins that we aim to ameliorate.

Gender in Core Human Archetypes

We now move on to explore four core human archetypes that we all share. Each culture that we come from shapes the way in which these archetypes appear to us, but they all spring from the same shared pool of psychological understanding.

The social conditioning of gender is a key factor. Every time we get up in the morning and dress according to our gender, we reinforce our belief in that gender. We have considerable expectations as to how the different genders will act. The difference was obvious when looking at traditional societies, but it is still very common today that indoor tasks are the remit of women, while outdoor tasks – especially those involving construction, repairs, or anything dangerous – tend to be in the male domain. More recent evolutionary developments are more malleable. We can change ideas easier than we can change biology.

Physical and emotional reactions are the most fixed and unchangeable, and social conventions are the most amenable to change. If we can change the language and the underlying feeling in society towards how gender and other aspects of life are, then we can change social conventions that will eventually impact on the archetypes. Today, there is a strong focus on alternative gender expressions and the more we choose to enable these alternative voices, the stronger they will become in our collective psyche.

Particularly in Western societies, the concept of gender has only recently been challenged. History has generally presented gender as binary. Nonbinary people have been either ignored or forgotten, and have been subjugated by patriarchal social structures (Zipes, 2012).

The following chapters examine four core archetypes: the king, the warrior, the magician, and the lover. It has been necessary to decide on the gender of these archetypes. This is not an easy choice, because whatever is chosen will highlight one way of seeing the world and exclude others, and whatever choices we make – particularly at the social level – will have consequences in our lives. It is important to keep this in mind. Should you choose to follow up and discover authors who have looked at other gendered arrangements of the archetypes, you may wish to read *The Heroine's Journey* (Murdoch, 2020), *The Hero Within* (Pearson, 1986), *The Goddess in Everywoman* (Bolen, 2009), and *Sage, Huntress, Lover, and Queen* (Branscombe, 2023).

Carl Jung (2014) wrote of the three archetypes of the king, the warrior, and the magician. Robert Moore and Douglas Gillette (1990) extended these to add a fourth core archetype: the lover. They conceived of these archetypes as all male.

As you will read, I have chosen to assign genders to each archetype, creating interesting patterns as the archetypes interact with one another. Please take these genders lightly. They shed light on the archetypes and make them more visible; but in doing so, other equally valid possibilities remain hidden.

Male and female roles have changed to become almost unrecognisable since archetypes were first established. Archetypes are slow to change because they are so deeply embedded in our psyche. With modern technology, so many of the differences between men and women have been overcome. Today, anyone can push a button to make something happen. Women have proven themselves to be totally capable in many realms of life that were previously closed to them. We see modern-day attempts to present women in mythological roles in different ways, such as Princess Leia in *Star Wars* and Dorothy in *The Wizard of Oz*. Characters in movies generally portray women in a different light from that in which they have been traditionally portrayed. There is still much more to be done. The tendency of archetypes to support the status quo is a significant hindrance to be addressed.

References

Bolen, JS (2009). *Goddesses in Everywoman: Powerful Archetypes in Women's Lives.* HarperOne.

Bowles, S (2009). The Emergence of Inequality and Hierarchy: A Network Explanation. Santa Fe Institute. https://sites.santafe.edu/~bowles/NetworkExplanation.pdf

Branscombe, M (2023). *Sage, Huntress, Lover, Queen: Access your Power and Creativity through Sacred Female Archetypes.* Findhorn Press.

Campbell, J (1991). *The Masks of God, Vol. 1: Primitive Mythology*. Penguin.

de Waal, FBM (2022). *Different: Gender through the Eyes of a Primatologist.* W W Norton & Co, Inc.

Debowska, A, Mattison, MLA, & Boduszek, D (2015). Gender Differences in the Correlates of Reactive Aggression. *Polish Psychological Bulletin, 46*(3), 469–476.

Dostoyevsky, F (2002). *The Brothers Karamazov.* Farrar, Strauss and Giraux.

Eisler, R (1988). *The Chalice and the Blade: Our History, Our Future.* HarperOne.

Farrell, W (1993). *The Myth of Male Power: Why Men are the Disposable Sex.* Simon& Shuster.

Fischer, AH, Rodrigeuz Mosquera, PM, & van Vianen, AEM (2004). Gender and Culture Differences in Emotion. *Emotion, 4*(1), 8794.

Freedman, EB (2002). *No Turning Back: The History of Feminism and the Future of Women.* Ballantine Books.

Gemes, K (2001). Postmodernism's Use and Abuse of Nietzsche. *Philosophy and Phenomenological Research, 62*(2), 337–360.

Graeber, D & Wengrow, D (2021). *The Dawn of Everything: A New History of Humanity.* Farrar, Strauss and Giruax.

Hodder, I (2006). *The Leopard's Tale: Revealing the Mysteries of Çatalhöyük.* Thames & Hudson.

Holy Bible, New King James Version (2018). Thomas Nelson.

Jung, C (2014). *The Archetypes and the Unconscious (Collected Works of C.G Jung)* (2nd Edition). Routledge.

Kanter, RM (1976). The Impact of Hierarchical Structures on the Work Behavior of Women and Men. *Social Problems, 23*(4), 415–430.

Lakoff, G (2014). Metaphor and War: The Metaphor System Used to Justify the War in the Gulf. *Peace Research, 23*(2), 25–32.

Manning, P (2023). Households and Communities: Evolution in Homo Sapiens. *The History of the Family*, *28*(4), 631–659.

Mäntylä, T (2013). Gender Differences in Multitasking Reflect Spatial Ability. *Psychological Science*, *24*(4), 514–520.

Mathias, P (2001). *The First Industrial Nation: The Economic History of Britain 1700–1914* (2nd Edition). Routledge.

Mead, HM (2016). *Tikanga Maori: Living by Maori Values* (Revised). Huia Publishers.

Melloni, A (ed). (2017). *Martin Luther: A Christian Between Reforms and Modernity (1517–2017)*. De Gruyter.

Moore, R & Gillette, D (1990). *King, Warrior, Magician, Lover*. Harper Collins.

Murdoch, M (2020). *The Heroine's Journey: Women's Quest for Wholeness*. Shambhalla.

Nietzsche, F (1883/1964). *Thus Spake Zarathustra: A Book for Everyone and No One* (1st Edition). Penguin.

Pearson, C (1986). *The Hero Within: Six Archetypes We Live By*. HarperSanFrancisco.

Politopoulos, A, Frieman, C, & Flexner, J (2024). An Anarchist Archaeology of Equality: Pasts and Futures Against Hierarchy. *Cambridge Archaeological Journal*, *34*(4), 531–544.

Real, T (1998). *I Don't Want to Talk About It: Overcoming the Secret Legacy of Male Depression*. (Reprint Edition). Scribner.

Ryali, S, Zhang, Y, Supekar, K, & Menon, V (2024). Deep Learning Models Reveal Replicable, Generalizable, and Behaviorally Relevant Sex Differences in Human Functional Brain Organization. *Proceedings of the National Academy*, *121*(9).

Schmidt, K (2010). Göbekli Tepe – The Stone Age Sanctuaries. New Results of Ongoing Excavations with a Special Focus on Sculptures and High Reliefs. *Documenta Praehistorica*, *37*, 239–256.

Schmidt Mast, M (2004). Men are Hierarchical, Women are Egalitarian: An Implicit Gender Stereotype. *Swiss Journal of Psychology*, *63*(2), 107–111.

Shaheen, U, Mumtaz, N, & Khalid, K (2019). Exploring Gender Ideology in Fairy Tales: A Critical Discourse Analysis. *International Journal of Academic Research*, *7*(3), 1–115.

Stoet, G, O'Connor, DB, Conner, M, & Laws, KR (2013). Are Women Better than Men at Multi-tasking? *BMC Psychology*, *1*(18).

Vervaeke, J (2019). *Awakening from the Meaning Crisis*. Youtube Video Series. youtube.com/watch?v=5418_ewcOIY

Wilber, K (2007). *A Brief History of Everything*. Shambhala Publications.

Wrangham, R (2019). *The Goodness Paradox: The Strange Relationship Between Virtue and Violence in Human Evolution*. Pantheon.

Zipes, J (2012). *The Irresistible Fairy Tale: The Cultural and Social History of a Genre*. Princeton University Press.

7 The King, Warrior, Magician, and Lover

Introduction

We now move to a new part of the journey. Having gained an understanding of archetypes and how they function, it is time to meet them. As we journey through our new land, we will encounter characters and interact with them. Ultimately, these prove to be parts of ourselves reflected back to us. They all have lessons to teach us about who we are and how we fit into our world. Some core characters have a significant influence over our lives.

As we evolved into human communities, we needed to communicate, which necessitated having sufficiently similar patterns in each of our minds to make sense of our world in a coherent and shareable way. The more we talked and interacted, the more these shared mental forms took on a life of their own within our collective psyche. As we already know, we developed social roles in our early traditional societies that made these communities more resilient and gave them advantages over communities that lacked such specialised roles. Four roles identified in traditional cultures worldwide have evolved into core archetypes, enabling us to act appropriately in our social roles.

The King

The earliest human groups were small family groups, in which everyone had a voice. Consensus decisions could generally be made with ease. As soon as a community reaches even 50 people, however, taking everyone's views into account becomes lengthy and unwieldy. Choosing a person or a small group to undertake that task on behalf of the whole group becomes far more efficient. Each community member cedes decision-making to the leader. Sometimes this person is chosen and sometimes the choice is forced onto the group. The leader must be able to contain their own entropy and that of the group. The larger the community, the more power accrues to the leader or leadership group. If the leader does not act competently or in the best interests of the people, they may find themselves removed from the leadership position.

The king is depicted as male, as throughout history, those in power have tended to be male. The king is also associated with rational thinking. As we work to redefine the

DOI: 10.4324/9781003675266-8

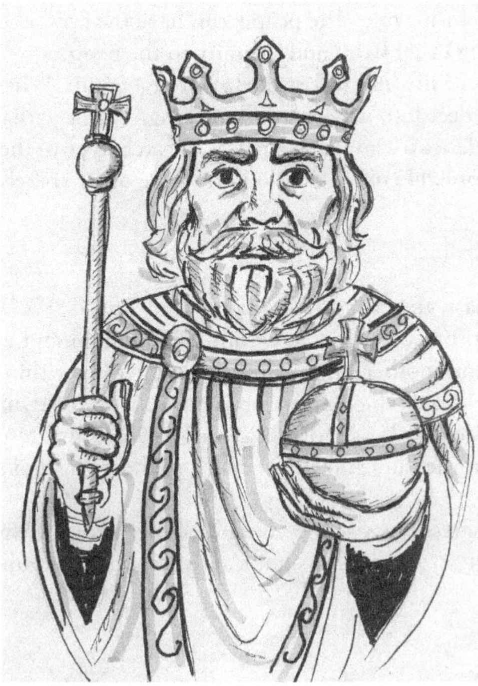

Figure 7.1 The king.

king in ways that are more relevant to today, we are reminded of the traditional archetype still alive within us, still shaping our behaviour.

In addition to supporters, there are always challengers. Each new decision leaves a space for opposition that the leader must manage. There is virtually always another potential leader waiting to assume the position. Typically, there are rewards for the person taking on the extra responsibilities, such as wealth and privilege. A wise ruler makes good decisions and retains the continued support of the people. However, some leaders are not wise. They make ill-advised decisions or ones that benefit them personally rather than the people. As a ruler sees themselves as losing control and power, they tend to slip into more coercive and controlling ways of leading. Often, the desire to maintain power leads to abusive and violent acts. We see the role of the king in the dynamics of life model (covered in Chapter 4) – first in the decision-making, which is a part of the 'making sense' process before acting; and second, in the emergent hierarchical levels.

The prime quality of the king is authority, which gives him the power to act. The king must act to ensure that all is well within the kingdom. The land must be bountiful, work must be coordinated, rules must be established and enforced, and relations with neighbouring kingdoms must be managed. The king creates order and predictability to prevent the kingdom from being overwhelmed by entropy.

The king is the figurehead that everyone respects and looks to for guidance. He must, therefore, act in ways that befit his role. The people can have the power to take back their authority should the king bring harm and calamity to the people.

The king is apparent at all levels of life, not just as the leader of a group. Whenever we take the initiative and make a decision, we act from our king. When parliament enacts a law or a child asserts their desire for an ice cream, it is the archetype of the king operating. The king cannot rule alone. He needs the support of the other archetypes.

The Warrior

The warrior is the one who hears the king's commands and enacts the king's proclamations. The warrior must protect the people within the kingdom and ensure that no harmful attacks come from another kingdom, or indeed from within. The quality of the warrior is courage, without which no action is possible. In the dynamics of life model, the warrior is the 'respond' part of sense, make sense, and respond. This archetype can also be found in the punishment functions of the living and social system.

In smaller communities, transgressions can be monitored by group members. However, as soon as the community size increases significantly, especially beyond the

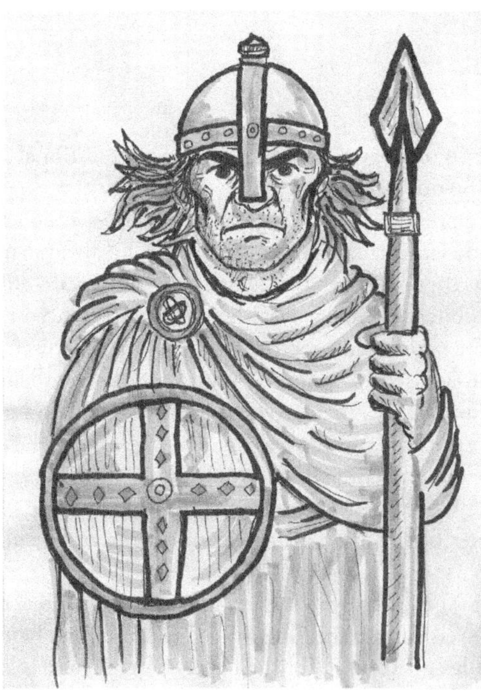

Figure 7.2 The warrior.

point where everyone knows each other, a more organised way of monitoring the group for transgressions is needed. A whole new specialised role is required.

The warrior protects the boundaries to ensure that no harm enters the kingdom. Our immune system patrols the body, searching for alien forms that may negatively impact our health. Threats from within the kingdom may also need to be managed.

The warrior is typically depicted as male and is often associated with courageous action. The warrior will withstand great hardship to do what is right. Any time we show courage in our lives and step into the unknown and unpredictable, we operate from our warrior. It is the police making an arrest or the drug addict choosing to stop using.

The Magician

The traditional leader acts as a figurehead but lacks the wisdom to make independent decisions. The leader needs a pool of wise people, such as elders or shamans, who hold the wisdom of the past, passed down from generation to generation. The quality of the magician is therefore wisdom. The wisdom holders also act as a check on the power of the leader. They can see when personal ambition might get the better of the leader or when their decisions are not well founded.

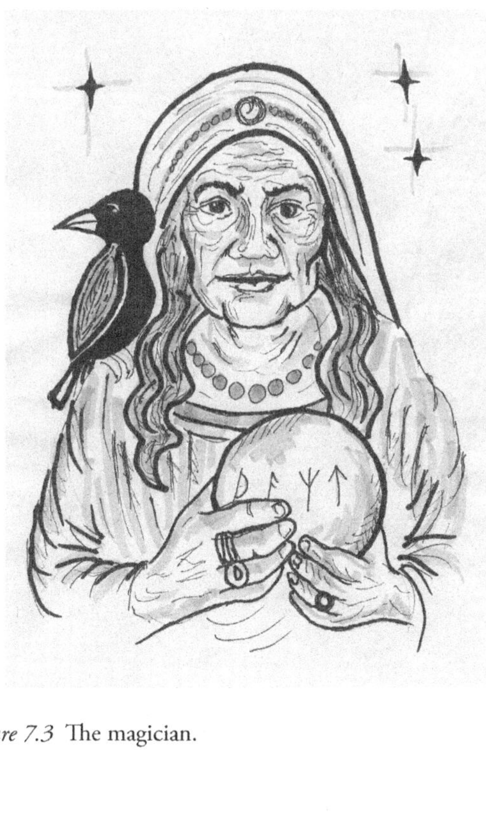

Figure 7.3 The magician.

Wisdom, as Sophia, has traditionally been female. She sees the bigger picture that the king might not see. Whereas the king must make definite black-and-white decisions, the magician inhabits a different, magical realm. Time and space are not fixed as they are for the king. There are links between the magician and the right brain, which manages functions that inhabit liminal realms beyond time and space and anything new and outside the box.

The Lover

Finally, there must be nurturers who care for the needs of the weaker or more vulnerable members of the community, such as children, older people, women, and the sick or injured. This links to the monitoring system of any living or social system, always seeking out parts that need help and support. They also ensure that the king does not have a cold heart but remains connected to the people and the kingdom. The legitimacy of the leader rests with the people. If they no longer choose to follow the king, the king becomes powerless. The nurturer is linked to the reward system, just as the warrior is connected to the punishment system. The lover is also female, linking to tasks of nurturing. Jung wrote about the anima and animus. The anima is the female aspect found within the male archetypes, while the animus is the male aspect within the female. Irrespective of gender, we are all a mix of male and female energies.

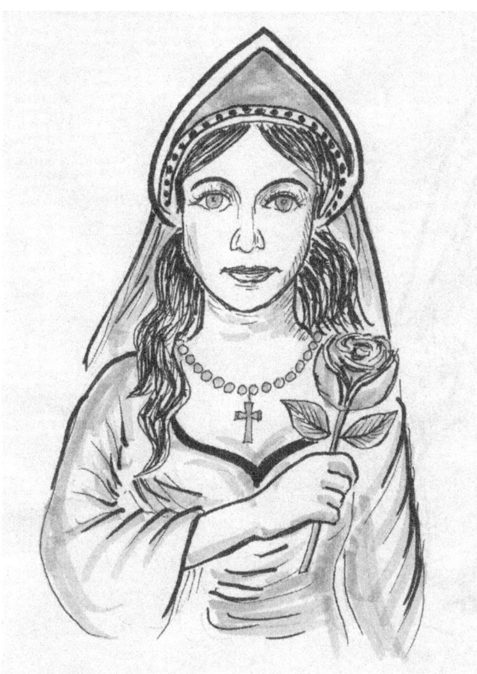

Figure 7.4 The Lover.

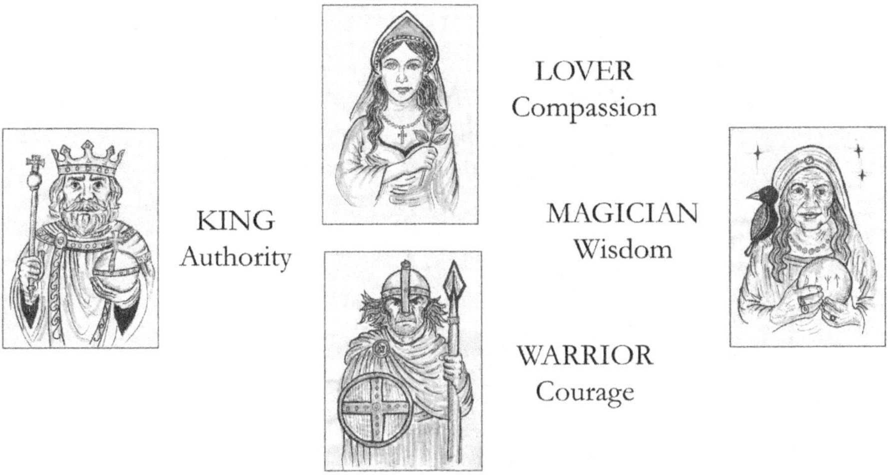

Figure 7.5 The king, the warrior, the magician, and the lover, and their associated qualities.

As shown in Figure 7.1, all four archetypes support and strengthen one another. They are interdependent, just as the different parts of the brain are interdependent, allowing us to function as a complete individual. They dwell as archetypes in the minds of all members of a society, reflecting key social roles and the core qualities of authority, courage, wisdom, and compassion. Any group member can use the archetype as a map of those roles to know how to attend to and respond to people fulfilling those roles in their community. For example, if I need a decision, I go to the king (eg, president, chairperson, team leader); if I need clarity, I go the magician; and if I need action, I turn to the warrior.

The Dragon

Whenever any of the four core archetypes falls out of balance, the dragon arises. The dragon represents those parts of ourselves that we are unwilling or unable to embrace. When we are overwhelmed by entropy, the dragon is given life. Sooner or later, we will meet the dragon on our journey. The parts that we reject become an external 'other' and can easily be turned into the enemy that we must fight or defeat; but there is always an 'other' within us that constellates as the dragon (Papadopoulos, 2006).

The dragon appears at all levels within us. We will face physical ailments if we fail to care for our bodies. If we suppress emotions, they lie hidden within, ready to appear at any time. If we distort our thinking, we end up with beliefs and values that will create undesired outcomes; and if we break social rules, we will face a social reaction.

When we are overwhelmed and unable to respond appropriately, we deny, minimise, blame, or justify how we make sense of the event to avoid facing it (Bandura, 1977). We push it away, back into the world; but we have already experienced the event, so it is already a part of us. Because we are unwilling or unable to embrace it, it

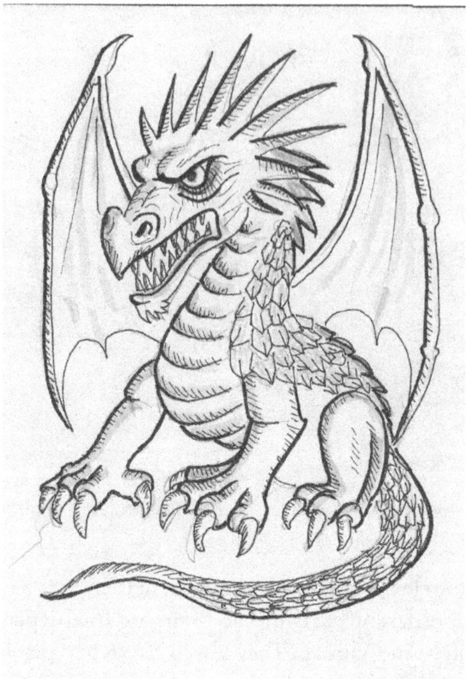

Figure 7.6 The dragon.

becomes unconscious. All these events constellate within as the dragon archetype. It is hidden away, growing stronger and stronger. While living in the castle, we are shielded from the dragon; but once we leave the castle and venture forth into life, the dragon lies in wait for our arrival. As we act in our lives, we create consequences for ourselves that we must later deal with.

The dragon is closely associated with the king, magician, warrior, and lover, and appears in some form in all fairytales. This may take the form of a demon, a goblin, a witch, a wizard, a serpent, or myriad other forms. As any core archetype moves out of balance by being either over-expressed or under-expressed, the dragon takes shape.

We fear the dragon because it appears as an obstacle to our lives. The dragon destroys and takes things from us. If we delve deeper into the dragon's nature, we see that it seeks healing. It is those parts of ourselves that we have denied and suppressed. When we have done things wrong, the dragon relentlessly points out our errors. It does not go away until errors are corrected.

I realised this while watching the third *Star Wars* movie, *The Return of the Jedi*. Luke Skywalker and the band of Jedi warriors enter the Cloud City. Obi-Wan Kenobi is in the middle of a duel with Darth Vader. Obi-Wan looks across and sees Luke. He knows that Luke has grown and learned enough to take over from him. Luke has internalised the wisdom of Obi-Wan. At this point, Obi-Wan raises his lightsabre, allowing Darth Vader to kill him, since he no longer needs to remain in his present form. This will enable Obi-Wan to transcend his self and take on an even stronger spiritualised form. Luke's journey must continue. He has integrated the positive side, but must next integrate his shadow.

Luke Skywalker later fatefully meets up with his nemesis in the form of Darth Vader, who we find out is Luke's father. Darth Vader was a Jedi warrior on the side of light but was seduced by the Emperor Palpatine into the powers of darkness. He has an evil, mechanical look – more machine than man. This has been the fate of so many men. Darth Vader has all but lost his humanity. Luke, an up-and-coming Jedi knight, now confronts him. While Luke and Darth Vader are divided, the Emperor has power. As they fight with lightsabres, Luke may be swayed by the powers of darkness and Darth Vader may return to the light. During the fight, Luke allows his hatred to surface, and as he does so, his hand is covered by a black glove. The dark side takes hold of him, but he notices this and centres himself. Darth Vader makes his choice and hurls the Emperor into the void of space. Luke and Darth Vader come together, so there is no space left for the Emperor to exist and he dies. At this point, the father and son are reunited. Luke can take off the mechanical mask and see his father as he truly is. Darth Vader then dies, because he too has become integrated back into Luke. Luke's shadow has been dissolved.

In *Facing the Dragon* (2003), Robert Moore suggests that the single-biggest reason why the dragon forms in people is grandiosity – that is, when people inflate themselves as more than they are. This happens when our map of ourselves grows out of proportion. We think that we are more important than we actually are. We all need to feel good about ourselves, what we do, and how others perceive us. When that feels threatened, one way in which we seek to combat this is by creating a false, larger-than-life image. That works well enough until we are inevitably challenged by an event in the world. Something will happen to contradict the map that we have of ourselves and our place in the world.

This sense of grandiosity often manifests as contempt and an unbalanced sense of entitlement, which gives 'permission' to act in ways that harm others. At other times, the pendulum swings to the opposite end: to a feeling of worthlessness and victimhood, where the dragon devours the person.

The 12 Archetypes

The further we explore the enchanted land, the more characters we meet. They do not always act as we would like them to. They have their own stories that have shaped them into who they are. As with the king, warrior, magician, and lover, these new characters have something to teach us about ourselves.

As a system is always less complex than the world in which it lives, no living system can know everything. It cannot always predict the future perfectly. Error is inherent in life. We all misjudge situations, often overreacting or underreacting to what is happening. We will perceive evil where it does not exist and overlook harmful circumstances. Since that is an inherent part of who we are, it will be reflected in the archetypes that inhabit us.

Error and evil are, therefore, not something external that attacks us and that we can identify and expel. Evil is eternally within us. It is baked into the pie from the beginning. It is so tempting to identify a scapegoat, within or without, to blame. Rather, we must come to terms with evil as a part of who we are.

For each of the four core archetypes, there is an over-expression and an under-expression. Including the four core archetypes creates a circle of 12 archetypes that form interesting patterns as they interact with each other. We will first examine each of the new archetypes and then explore how they interact.

The Tyrant

The tyrant is the archetype of the over-expressed king. The king's quality is authority. When the king's authority is used to control and manipulate others in harmful ways, this is damaging and destructive. It is usually intended to boost the tyrant's ego. The tyrant has forgotten that they only have the authority they do because it has been invested in them through the people.

The tyrant has come to feel that he cannot meet his needs through the proper expression of authority and falls back on political manoeuvring and exploitation to get

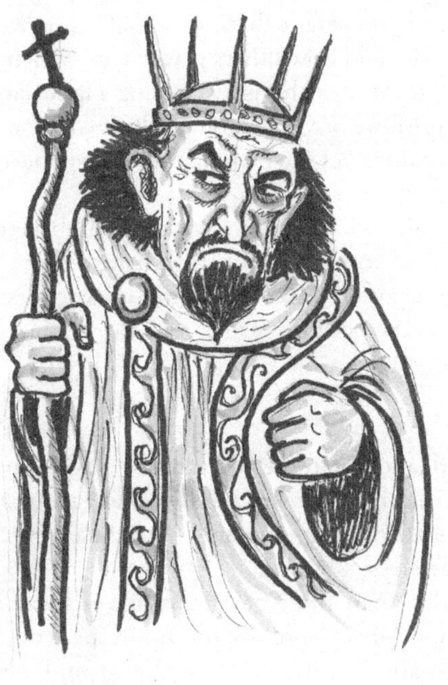

Figure 7.7 The tyrant.

what he wants. The tyrant will use his power and resources for his own needs rather than those of the people, who will suffer at his hands. The tyrant usually works hard to maintain an image that the people will believe in; but behind the mask, the tyrant is more concerned about himself than his people. History is filled with tyrants who caused havoc in the lives of their people.

The Clown

The clown is the under-expression of the king. This is the king who is unwilling or unable to exert his sense of authority. The clown is clumsy and inept. His clothes are gaudy and inappropriate. The king needs to be a resolute figurehead that people can have confidence in to act on their behalf, but the clown cannot do this. People laugh at his ineptitude.

There is an interesting variant of the clown in the jester. The jester sits at court and pokes fun at all the characters and social agreements that the king has been selected to represent. Nobody else dares to make fun of the king or his high station. If the king has become too rigid in how he wields his authority, the jester is often the only person who can make those cutting remarks that point out the ultimate lack of foundation of the king's power. However, the jester must be careful not to go too far, or he too might lose his head. The tyrant or the clown arises when the king fails to project his

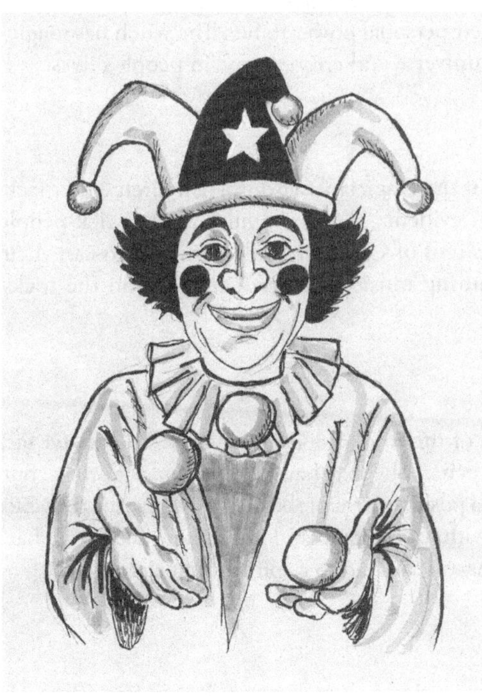

Figure 7.8 The clown.

sense of authority appropriately. Often this is because the king has stopped listening to the other core archetypes that can support him in areas where his qualities might be lacking.

The Bully

The bully is the overexpression of the warrior. The warrior is the one who acts. The warrior must protect those in his care; but as the bully, he misuses his physical advantage to force others to conform to his desires. The bully also does not obey the king or heed the advice and warnings of the other archetypes. The bully must have his own way, irrespective of what that might mean for other people.

The Coward

The coward is the under-expression of the warrior. The coward lacks the warrior's courage to stand and do what is needed. He runs and hides right when he needs to stand and be firm. He fails the very people whom he is charged to protect.

The Witch

The witch is the over-expression of the wisdom of the magician or wise person. Wisdom is manipulated for personal gain. The witch tells lies and tricks people into incorrect beliefs, persuading them to give their personal power to her. The witch has magic spells that break the normal flow of the universe and create havoc in people's lives.

The Siren

The siren is the under-expression of the magician's wisdom. The siren either lacks that wisdom or chooses not to make it evident. The siren will lure and trick people into doing what she wants, just as the sirens of Greek mythology sought to cast their spell on Odysseus through their enchanting music and wreck his ship on the rocks. The siren is manipulative and devious.

The Martyr

The martyr is the under-expression of the compassion of the lover. The martyr sacrifices herself for others, but at her own expense. She may have compassion for others, but lacks it for herself. Like the jester, there is a positive form of the martyr, where she truly sacrifices herself for others; but this is done without coercion and in full knowledge of what she is doing. The true expression of the martyr can lead to a spiritual transformation.

The Overprotective Mother

The overprotective mother uses compassion to smother and manipulate others, thereby gaining control over them. This denies them the freedom to fulfil the potential within them. She acts to meet her own needs.

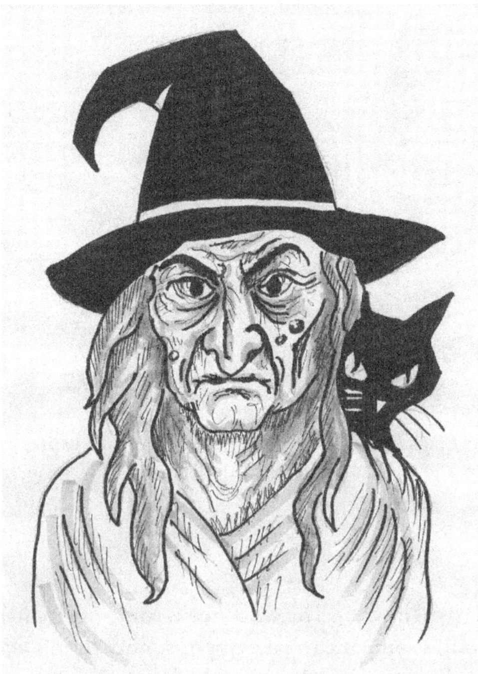

Figure 7.9 The witch.

We can see how the 12 archetypes fit together in Figure 7.10.

The Interactions between the Archetypes

There are patterns that arise between these archetypes, where the over-expressed archetype is attracted to the under-expressed archetype on the opposite side of the diagram. Let us start with the tyrant and the siren.

The Tyrant and the Siren

The tyrant seeks to control everyone, including his partner. He does not want an intelligent person who might challenge him or make him look silly in front of others. The tyrant is concerned with his image and wants someone whose attractiveness will appeal to others.

The siren is the manipulative partner. She will play along with the tyrant because she thinks that her needs will be met through his power. If she is intelligent, she may manipulate him to gain power for herself. The siren uses her sexuality as a weapon to get what she wants.

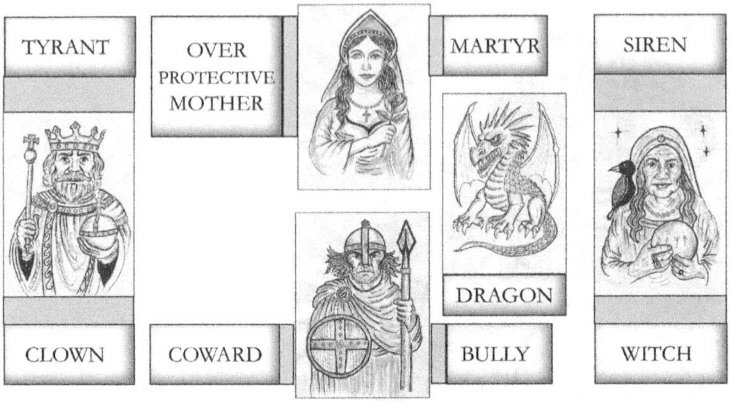

Figure 7.10 The king, the warrior, the magician, and the lover, with the over-expressed and under-expressed archetypes and the dragon in the middle.

The Witch and the Clown

The witch and the clown are drawn to each other. The witch seeks someone to manipulate and control, while the clown desires someone to take responsibility for his actions. The clown feels incompetent and seeks someone who seems to have the wisdom he is looking for, but is equally wounded. He naturally finds that he cannot meet the witch's standards, and she becomes bitter and angry as a result. The witch's anger scares the clown, who feels stressed and thus even less competent, and is constantly afraid of criticism and rejection. This can turn into a destructive downward spiral in which fear and incompetence form a destructively amplifying positive feedback loop.[1] This situation worsens increasingly until the relationship ends. The clown needs to take responsibility and stand up, while the witch needs to learn to accept. Only then might they return to the balance of the king and the wise person. The story of Blimpo the Clown (Appendix I) explores these two archetypes.

A man living through the clown archetype will feel clumsy and incompetent, especially if attacked by the witch. The clown may choose to stonewall, frozen by the fear of being attacked, which may be genuine. It feels better to do nothing and say nothing, but that further enrages the witch. The clown may try to deflect by turning everything into a joke. The witch will ridicule and denigrate, nag and complain. She will gaslight and deceive, blame and vilify.

The Bully and the Martyr

The bully seeks someone to control and the martyr sacrifices herself, often believing that the bully will change and return to being a warrior. However, her passive acceptance of his aggression makes her more entrapped. Courage and compassion have been lost, and only through genuine expressions of courage and compassion can this relationship dynamic return to being expressions of the warrior and lover.

The warrior will threaten, intimidate and use violence to get his way. The bully controls through fear; while the martyr hides away, hiding her pain.

The Overprotective Mother and the Coward

The overprotective mother cannot meet her own needs in herself and regains her feeling of control by taking over the coward. The coward lacks the courage to break free and create his own life; while the overprotective mother lacks the compassion and empathy to recognise and address the suffocating impact of her actions. She stunts the growth of the coward, so he never finds out who he is but is always at her beck and call.

Whenever archetypes are out of balance, dysfunction arises and harm is experienced. All that cannot be resolved and managed by the core archetypes gives power to the dragon to grow and devour.

Note

1 A positive feedback loop is one where a quality of the system gets larger and larger. In this case, the anger grows with an increasingly negative outcome. A negative feedback loop keeps a system in the same state, like a thermostat.

Bibliography

Bandura, A (1977). *Social Learning Theory* (1st Edition). Prentice Hall.

Moore, RL (2003). *Facing the Dragon: Confronting Personal and Spiritual Grandiosity.* Chiron Publications.

Papadopoulos, RK (2006). *The Handbook of Jungian Psychology: Theory, Practice and Applications.* Routledge.

8 *The Wizard of Oz*

Introduction

We have encountered many characters on our journey that reveal our inner nature. The archetypes reflect the processes within us as we move through our lives. We have told stories ever since we first sat together around a campfire. As the archetypes interact, they create stories that unfold over time. These archetypes came to life in the flickering flames and the whistling wind. Archetypes took shape in the stars. Each story arises from a particular culture with its own way of seeing the world.

The stories are expressed through different media. From storytelling, we have dance and drama. Particularly today, new formats such as films give us much more flexibility in how we share archetypal stories.

As we make our way through life, we pass through different stages. These are not strict, linear stages, one following another, and each person's pathway through life will be individual; but there are general patterns that can help to illuminate and make sense of the events in our lives.

We follow the basic themes of being born, followed by a time of innocent childhood. For some, this childhood does not last long – they are thrust into the adult world before their time. We grow into adulthood learning the skills that we need to operate as citizens within the culture or cultures in which we are raised. We tend to form families, pursue careers, and establish ourselves in our communities. There will be good times and bad, and obstacles to overcome. We will suffer loss and hardship.

We will pass our peak times at the various levels of our being. Our physical abilities will decline, requiring us to readjust our lives. We will take on numerous roles, from child to parent to grandparent. Death awaits us all. It may come early in our journey or in later decades. Different cultures understand the stages differently, but there are underlying patterns that are useful to explore.

We have already encountered the hero's journey woven through many traditional fairytales and myths. Great wisdom is encoded in all the elements of a fairytale or myth, revealing much about human nature. Fairytales and myths are distilled down to their barest elements to make them memorable, so no detail is superfluous.

The word 'myth', interestingly, has two meanings. The first is an untrue story; the second is a story from ancient times describing the history of the people and how

DOI: 10.4324/9781003675266-9

the present world came to be. Myths arose from the stories that people told each other about their lives. Over time, the exploits of individuals were exaggerated and embellished to add intensity and effect to a story.

As we became self-conscious as human beings, we came to realise that we would die one day. We had not previously realised this in such a stark way. A fear arose about our personal future and what happens after death. We needed to rethink how to find value and purpose in our lives. We created stories to answer the big questions of where we came from and where we would go when we die. These give us hope and solace to stave off the angst of the meaninglessness of life.

This means that we need stories that make sense of the world we live in and help us to navigate the trials and tribulations of life. Our ancestors spent countless nights under the stars sitting around a fire telling stories that could be distilled down to an essence that embodied the fullness of the existential challenges before us. The stories needed to be simple enough to be passed down successfully from generation to generation. Each culture found its own pathway.

A Guide to Revealing Meaning in Fairytales

Fairytales and myths have typically been remembered by heart, especially in societies without written forms. They have been passed down through generations. The stories have been trimmed back to mere essentials, so that everything has meaning. Each element in a story is a part of who we are. We are each of the archetypes. Not only the characters but also the objects in the story – with their colours, shapes, and textures – all have meaning. The time of day could reflect a stage that has been reached. Male objects are typically long and thin, such as a sword or a pillar; while female objects are often containers, such as a cup or an oven.

It is also revealing to look at who is present and who is absent. Cinderella's mother died and her father remarried a proud, haughty woman with two daughters. The stepmother is jealous of Cinderella. This is therefore the story of a young woman being brought up without a caring, motherly influence. Hansel and Gretel live with a woodsman who has a second wife, who proposes that the children be abandoned in the woods because they are too poor to care for them. Jack and the Beanstalk is a story about a boy brought up without a father. The giant represents the shadow that arose for Jack as he lived without a father.

The elements of nature – fire, air, earth, and water – can have symbolic meaning. Apples are often seen as forbidden fruit that leads to loss. A mirror reflects the truth back to the person looking in. Shoes can symbolise being set free to move forward; and lanterns or torches represent a lighted way forward that banishes darkness. The sea is often a symbol of the unconscious, so any fish or creature emerging from the sea is an unconscious aspect becoming conscious.

Often, the original stories have been watered down or Disneyfied so that some of the cruelty and violence are removed. While this is understandable, given that today children are the main audience for fairytales, there is also a loss. The dragon is made less frightening. This can lead us to dismiss the power of the dragon to devour us – and it will devour us if we are not firm enough with it. In the story of Cinderella, the two ugly sisters cut off parts of their feet to try to fit into the shoe that the prince has found. They are found out because their blood flows out onto the bottom of the carriage as they travel back to the castle. At the end of the story, birds come down and peck out their eyes as punishment for their evil deeds.

The Wizard of Oz film removed some of the more gruesome acts of violence from the original book.

With this knowledge in our magic bag, we are ready to examine a selection of fairytales and myths from around the world, exploring the hidden meanings that can guide us on our own hero's journey.

The Wizard of Oz

The Wizard of Oz is a remarkable story by L Frank Baum (1900/2000), first published in 1900, which exemplifies the journey of life as a journey through the magical land of Oz. Some versions of the book use the title *The Wonderful Wizard of Oz*. Baum was born and raised in New York. He loved theatre and writing from a young age. He moved to South Dakota, which inspired the background setting of the story in Kansas.

When the book was published, it became an instant success. L Frank Baum and others also turned it into a musical. Significant changes to the storyline may have been influenced by other people's ideas rather than Baum's choice. The stage version was called *The Wizard of Oz*, a title which was retained for the film. The film was not an instant success, but it gained popularity in the 1950s.

L Frank Baum had a colourful life, marked by many successes and failures. He dabbled in religion and politics and was a controversial figure. He died after a stroke in 1919 at the age of 63. He was brought up as a Methodist but later became a Theosophist. Theosophy encompasses an esoteric set of beliefs. It draws heavily from Buddhism and Hinduism, which influenced the characters and plot of the story. Baum wrote many stories about Dorothy and the land of Oz, but the first book in particular exemplifies fairytale themes. Some of his later works were driven more by the need to make money to pay debts and do not have the same depth as his earlier works.

Most people are familiar with the story of *The Wizard of Oz* from the 1939 film adaptation. There are some significant differences between the book and the film. The film, in particular, adds more detail before Dorothy arrives in the land of Oz; and the book recounts other adventures, particularly after the Wizard of Oz has left in his balloon.

The story is set on a farm in Kansas during the Great Depression. Dorothy Gale, the heroine, is an orphan who is being brought up by her Aunt Em and Uncle Henry. At the time, such arrangements were much more common than today. Dorothy tries to be obedient and to do what is expected of her, but – like all children – she sometimes finds this hard and gets in trouble.

In Kansas, Dorothy lives in a sheltered world of innocence. She remains within the castle. She can only dream as far as the world about her. She is protected by her aunt and uncle, who are portrayed as stern and preoccupied with keeping everything running on the farm. There are hints of things to come in the storm clouds that approach. In the film, we meet the farmhands Hunk, who becomes the Scarecrow in the land of Oz; Hickory, the Tin Woodsman; and Zeke, the Cowardly Lion. When Dorothy falls into the pig enclosure, Zeke is the one with enough courage to leap in and get her out.

Hunk advises Dorothy to keep away from neighbour Myra Gulch. Myra wants to have Dorothy's dog, Toto, put down because he annoys her. Aunt Em and Uncle Henry are powerless to stop Myra from using the law to have Toto put down. Myra takes Toto away, but he escapes and returns to Dorothy. Myra becomes the Wicked Witch of the West. Dorothy decides to run away with Toto when she hears that Toto will be put down and encounters Professor Marvel, a travelling snake oil salesman, in his wagon as he moves from town to town. Professor Marvel hears Dorothy's story of running away and uses his glass ball to convince her to return home. None of this is in the book, but it allows for an interesting connection between the everyday world of Kansas and the magical land of Oz. Everything in Kansas is described as being dull and grey. The house is grey, with no green grass or trees. Even the people are described as grey. Only Toto is black. Toto can be seen as representing Dorothy's sense of intuition. He always does things that are not expected, which turn out to be just what is needed.

In the book, we are simply informed of a tornado approaching. Dorothy's innocence is about to end. She is unable to reach the underground shelter in time, so she is trapped inside the house when the tornado arrives. Some heroes get to choose their adventure, while others are thrust into a new world. Dorothy does not get the choice, just as Luke Skywalker has no choice after stormtroopers kill his uncle and aunt.

Suddenly, everything familiar disappears as Dorothy is swept up and taken across the threshold into a new land. Our young heroine leaves the old world to arrive in a new one. This is accentuated in the film by the sepia-coloured scenes in Kansas suddenly blooming into full Technicolor as soon as Dorothy sets foot in the land of Oz.

The Land of Oz

The farmhouse that Dorothy and Toto were in is sucked into the tornado and flies away, eventually landing in Oz – the home of the Munchkins, who have been terrorised by a wicked witch. Unbeknown to Dorothy, the house has landed on the Wicked Witch of the East and killed her. The Munchkins recognise Dorothy as a good witch who has the power to release them from bondage.

The Munchkins are dwarf-sized people about the same size as Dorothy. They are happy and cheerful. These small people might represent the fragmented nature of the young sense of self. A consistent sense of self has not yet developed. There is a movement back and forth between the many reflections of self. The Munchkins lack the courage to embark on the journey of personal growth. They remain in their bubble, growing older but not growing up to be adults. But this makes them vulnerable to harmful elements in the world, and thus they fell victim to the Wicked Witch of the East.

The Witch of the North visits the Munchkins to foreshadow what might be possible for Dorothy. She exclaims that Dorothy is small, like the Munchkins, and thus could never have been powerful enough to defeat the Wicked Witch of the East intentionally. She calms the frightened Munchkins and tells Dorothy that because she killed the Wicked Witch of the East, she can claim the silver slippers that the witch had been wearing. In the film, the witches of the North and South are combined into one character, named Glinda, which in the book is the name of the Witch of the South. Also, in the film, the silver slippers become ruby slippers because these looked more impressive in Technicolor.

Dorothy does not know it, but she is a good witch in training. She is given the silver slippers previously belonging to the Wicked Witch of the East. They are hers to claim and have magical powers that could help Dorothy. She does not put them on immediately. She later chooses them over the shoes that she was wearing because they will be better for the long journey.

However, Dorothy lacks the confidence to act as a good witch. As we later find out, she has the ability to return to Kansas through the slippers all along. In the same way, we are already complete and whole in our incompleteness, but we do not realise it. We all think that something is missing which, if we only had it, would make everything all right. Buddhism teaches us that nirvana is already with us in samsara; Jesus reminds us that the kingdom of heaven is at hand; and Mohammad says that Allah is closer to a person than their jugular vein.

The Yellow Brick Road and Dorothy's Companions

Dorothy wants to know how to return home and is told to go to Emerald City via the Yellow Brick Road and visit the Wizard of Oz there – he will surely know how she can get back to Kansas. Dorothy has courage that the Munchkins lack. She is willing to venture forth into an unknown world to get back home. Dorothy and Toto set forth on the Yellow Brick Road – a symbol for the journey of life – towards the Emerald City. The Witch of the North promises to guard and protect Dorothy on her journey – just as Obi-Wan Kenobi in *Star Wars* is always close by, helping and supporting Luke Skywalker on his journey. The witch gives Dorothy a protective kiss, which leave a visible mark, and then departs.

The favourite colour in Munchkinland is blue. It can be found everywhere. Even Dorothy's clothing is blue and white. Dorothy learns from a Munchkin that only witches can wear white. From the grey world of Kansas, we have moved into a blue world. It is different and marvellous, but Dorothy has yet to experience the full range of colours that would indicate a full life. The blue colours are not used explicitly in the film – presumably because they would not showcase the power of Technicolor.

Before long, Dorothy comes across the Scarecrow in a field and is surprised to discover that he can talk. The Scarecrow is stuffed with straw. Dorothy helps the Scarecrow down and he explains to her that he does not have a brain. The Scarecrow represents Dorothy's thinking and analytical mind, which at this point is undeveloped. He has a blue hat and his eyes are painted blue. Dorothy suggests that the Wizard of Oz might be able to help him, too, and invites him to join her on her journey as a companion. At first, Toto is suspicious of this new traveller. The intuitive mind and the rational mind perceive the world in vastly different ways. The Scarecrow represents the latent king waiting to develop thinking and analytical skills to make good decisions.

The Scarecrow is filled with straw, so he moves clumsily, reminiscent of a clown – an aspect of the king.

The Scarecrow was placed in the field by a farmer to scare away the crows. But one crow was smart enough to realise that the Scarecrow was not a Munchkin and started eating the corn, and other crows quickly followed. The crow spoke to the Scarecrow and told him that the only difference between him and a Munchkin was that he did not have a brain. This reminds us of the story of Adam and Eve. The serpent is portrayed as the evil character in the Bible, but it actually tells the truth. Without the serpent, Adam and Eve would be stuck in their innocent paradise forever, never knowing good and evil. The serpent tells them that they will not die if they eat the apple but will become like God. They do not die and become conscious of good and evil. Once their eyes have been opened to good and evil, the knowledge of death enters the world. Our journey of knowingly living through time and space, from birth to death, can only happen because the serpent told the truth. The crows similarly came and told the Scarecrow that he could learn and become fully human. The Scarecrow's only weakness is that a lighted match could burn him up. Each part of us will also have its own strengths and weaknesses.

The buildings at the beginning of Dorothy's journey through Oz are bright and cheerful. However, as she walks along the Yellow Brick Road, they lose some of their brightness. The houses are not cared for as they were at the beginning. As we begin the journey of life, everything is positive and exciting; but every now and then, an event happens that darkens the original, innocent dream.

Dorothy and the Scarecrow soon enter a dark, foreboding forest. There, she meets the Tin Woodsman, who tells her that he does not have a heart, and that he has become all rusted up and cannot move or cry. The Tin Woodsman, of course, represents Dorothy's heart – her connection to her emotions of love and compassion. As with the Scarecrow, the heart is not yet developed because she has had no interactions in the real world where, as an adult, she must suffer the consequences of her actions. The Tin Woodsman tells a story of falling in love with a Munchkin. He wanted to get married, but the Munchkin's mother did not want her to leave because she did all the work around the house. The mother went to a witch, who put a spell on the man by enchanting his axe. He ended up cutting off all his limbs, which were replaced by tin; but his heart could not be replaced and he lost his love for the Munchkin. We all have a story of our first love or an early love that did not last. We were probably just too young. We gave our hearts to someone else, which caused us to get hurt and hide our hearts to avoid getting wounded again. The Tin Woodsman's weakness is that his tin can rust, but he carries an oil can to prevent this from happening.

A little further down the road, Dorothy comes across a timid Lion with no courage. He tries to scare the group of travellers so that he can feel courageous. He attacks the Scarecrow and the Tin Woodsman and growls at Toto. Dorothy rushes in, grabs Toto, and hits the Lion on the nose. The Lion acknowledges that he is a coward and only scares people so that they won't notice he is a coward. This, then, is Dorothy's sense of courage, which will grow as they move deeper into the land of Oz.

The characters all seem as though they lack something important, just as Dorothy lacks the confidence to act as a good witch. All these capacities are latent within us, to be honed through our interactions in our daily lives. We also notice that all the characters display the attributes that they think they do not have. The Scarecrow often devises a plan of action. The Tin Woodsman shows compassion, even to a beetle that he accidentally treads on. (He weeps, showing compassion; but his tears cause him to rust and his jaws clamp up. The Scarecrow mindfully notices and gets the oil can to fix his jaw.) The Lion exhibits daring and courage on numerous occasions. As is often true with us, we often display the attributes that we think we lack, but either do not notice or choose to downplay them.

You will have noticed how Dorothy's companions match the four archetypes that we explored in the previous chapter. The Scarecrow links to the authority of the king to make clear, decisive decisions. Toto links to the wisdom of the magician. The Cowardly Lion represents the warrior's courage; and the Tin Woodsman represents the lover who has lost the ability to feel love and compassion. They will all accompany Dorothy as she ventures through the land of Oz. Their adventures and interactions will build each of them. They must support and help one another, just as the four core archetypes are interconnected and must collaborate and remain balanced for the optimal functioning of the whole self.

The four are now ready to continue down the Yellow Brick Road. They have begun to experience life as adults, rising to meet the challenges that they encounter. They have many adventures along the Yellow Brick Road. As they cross a great ditch by walking along a tree that the Tin Woodsman has cut down to serve as a bridge, they are chased by ugly monsters called Kalidahs. The Scarecrow yells out to the Tin Woodsman to cut the tree away once they have crossed the ditch, so that the Kalidahs fall off the tree and down onto the jagged rocks below. This part of the story is not included in the film.

They soon arrive at a river that they must cross. They decide to build a raft and all goes well until they reach the middle of the river, where the current is too strong. The raft is swept downstream towards the land of the Wicked Witch of the West. The Scarecrow's pole, which he has been using to try to steady the raft, gets stuck in the mud on the riverbed – with the Scarecrow still clinging onto it. As he has not yet developed his thinking skills, he is left trapped in the river.

The Lion suggests that he swim to the bank while they hold onto his tail. They manage to get the raft to the bank in this way but they are now far from the Yellow Brick Road. As we experience both good times and bad on our life's journey, we often get pulled away from our purpose and end up somewhere we had not intended. The travellers start out on the long journey back to the Yellow Brick Road until they reach the Scarecrow, still clinging for his life to the pole in the middle of the river. They do not know how to rescue him, but then, unexpectedly, a stork flies by. As the Scarecrow is only made of straw and is thus very light, the stork agrees to rescue him. Life may seem like a random set of events, but underlying patterns exist. If we can live our lives in harmony with the world that we are in, natural patterns can arise in seemingly magical ways to help us cope with otherwise impossible situations. I have noticed times when, unexpectedly, precisely what I needed appeared in my life at exactly the right time. At times, I did not recognise the seeming coincidence. If the world is fractal, harmonic patterns draw us towards wholeness. Joseph Campbell (1988) wrote,

'If you do follow your bliss, you put yourself on a kind of track that has been there all the while waiting for you, and the life that you ought to be living is the one you are living.'

As they all walk together back towards the Yellow Brick Road, they come across fields of flowers of all types and colours. This episode is included in the film. The scarlet poppies grow increasingly numerous. They have an enticing smell, especially when they are more abundant. Dorothy, Toto, and the Lion – all living creatures – feel drowsy and start to sleep. The Scarecrow and the Lion try to keep everyone moving before it gets dark. They pick up Dorothy and Toto and carry them, but the Lion is too heavy to lift.

As we journey through life, we can get caught up in the routine and become drowsy about keeping on with what really matters. Caring for children, paying the mortgage, advancing careers, building a house, and so many other necessary things to do in life blind us to the purpose that we held to when we started out on our own Yellow Brick Road. Many people never awaken from their sleep and die with their true song unsung within them. The film simplifies the metaphor. Instead of Dorothy awakening through her own inner clarity, the cause and solution are externalised: the Wicked Witch causes the sleep, while Glinda's snow breaks the spell.

According to the book, with the Lion left behind, the others move on. A great yellow wildcat chases a mouse right next to them. The Tin Woodsman raises his axe and cuts the head off the wildcat. Baum is no Walt Disney, cutting out the gory details. He knows that we can only respond to life's challenges if we are willing to see them as they are. The mouse, whose life is saved, turns out to be the queen of all the fieldmice. When other mice arrive, they offer to do anything that the Tin Woodsman wants. The Scarecrow suggests that the mice might help them save the Lion, who is still sleeping in the poppies.

The Scarecrow asks the Tin Woodsman to build a trolley out of wood to drag the Lion out of the poppy field. All the mice are asked to bring some string and thousands of mice together pull the Lion away from the flowers.

The Emerald City

Before long, the travellers find their way back to the Yellow Brick Road. Now, all the buildings are green. They soon reach the walls of the Emerald City. This is the boundary between the ordinary world and the special or sacred place. Unless someone has learned the necessary life lessons, they cannot be allowed to enter the holiest of holy spaces. It is unsafe for them to enter, as they would defile the holy space. Dorothy is allowed to enter the Emerald City; but often, there is a test at the threshold, so that only those who are prepared may enter. In the film, it is only once the Guardian of the Gates sees Dorothy's silver slippers that the doors are opened. In the book, they also notice the mark from the kiss of the good witch on her forehead.

If you enter a Buddhist temple, you will see a statue of a fierce demon on each side of the gateway and you must walk between them (Bocking, 1997). They represent the dualities of life. Buddhism advocates for the middle way, where we avoid falling into the temptation of making one side right and the other wrong but instead stay on the middle path – much like a tightrope walker who can walk forward by balancing the extremes.

On entering the Emerald City, they meet a Munchkin-sized man dressed in green. Everything is brighter, so everyone must wear green-coloured glasses because the light is so bright. Everything is hyper-real; but it is still only in one colour, so it is still only seeing life from one perspective. The glasses are not included in the film. This is part of the wizard's deception. Although he has no malicious intent, he wants to make people happy, but he tries to do this by shielding them from the unbearable truth. The film adds a horse which changes colour regularly. This symbolises the ability to look beyond one colour and see the world in full colour.

Nobody they encounter has ever seen the wizard. They say that he can take many forms. The group are brought into the wizard's palace and a soldier goes to inform the wizard, who is behind a curtain, of their arrival. They are instructed to visit the wizard one at a time. When Dorothy comes in, she finds that the wizard is just a big head and a booming voice. This symbolises the wizard's intelligence and the risk that Dorothy might focus excessively on the head over the heart. He asks how she came by the silver slippers and about the kiss mark on her forehead. Dorothy asks to be returned to Kansas. The wizard says that she must first kill the Wicked Witch of the West. In the film, this process is condensed into a single meeting with the wizard. Dorothy is instructed to return with the witch's broom. Dorothy does not want to kill anything, but the wizard insists.

As soon as we start out on the pathway of life, our actions have consequences. Dorothy's shadow of emotions, arising from everything that she has been unwilling or unable to manage, has been growing steadily over time. We must face up to our past. We must see and recognise the harm, both intentional and unintentional, that we have caused and release it. We must kill the dragon.

When the others meet with the wizard, he appears differently to each of them. He appears to the Scarecrow as a lovely lady dressed in green, representing the compassion that he risks lacking in his search for a brain. The Tin Woodsman encounters a terrifying beast, the size of an elephant, symbolising the consequences of unchecked emotions. The Lion sees a great ball of fire that is fearsome and may thwart the development of his courage. In the film, this idea of the wizard's shifting identities is handled differently. Instead of appearing in different forms, the film signals his constructed, performative power by having actor Frank Morgan play multiple roles: the guard at the city gate; the soldier at the palace; the driver of the horse of a different colour; Professor Marvel; and the wizard himself. His repeated presence hints that the wizard's authority is a matter of costume and performance rather than genuine transformation.

The Wicked Witch of the West

The party leave the Emerald City, following the setting sun, to arrive in the land of the Wicked Witch of the West. In the book, the witch only has one eye; but in the film, she has two. Dorothy's dress is now all white, rather than blue and white, and the ribbon around Toto's neck becomes all white, signifying her progression towards becoming a full good witch.

As soon as they arrive in the land, the Wicked Witch calls her pack of wolves. She decides that the travellers are not worth keeping as slaves, so she instructs the wolves to tear them apart. As the wolves attack, the Tin Woodsman kills them with his axe while Dorothy sleeps safely inside a little house that they have built for her. This illustrates the temptation of Christ, when the devil came to him, offering him power and riches if he would abandon his quest for truth. The Buddha sat beneath the bodhi tree, meditating. All manner of demons attacked him. The suppressed emotions of our lifetime rear up out of fear to protect themselves and attack, hoping that we will be frightened by their appearance and will return to live in the familiar fear. Behind the fear is a desire for healing. If we dare to hold fast when the apparitions of our past rise and rage, they will be seen for what they are.

The Tin Woodsman has developed his capacity for empathy and compassion and will protect those to whom he feels a strong attachment. We are left with the paradox that he is very concerned about stepping on a beetle by mistake but will willingly cut off the heads of many wolves. When the danger has passed, Dorothy wakes and steps outside, unaware of how fiercely her friends have protected her. Seeing all her wolves lying dead, the Witch sends a large flock of crows to attack the travellers. This time, it is the Scarecrow who scares the crows away. Those he does not scare, he grabs and strangles.

In all, 40 crows and 40 wolves are killed. This number is significant in the Bible and represents a time of trial or testing. The Israelites spent 40 years in the desert with Moses. Noah's flood lasted 40 days. Jesus spent 40 days in the desert, being tempted by the devil.

The witch next sends a plague of bees to attack the travellers. The Scarecrow sacrifices his straw to cover the Lion, Dorothy, and Toto so that they do not get stung; while the Tin Woodsman fights off the bees because their stings cannot penetrate his tin. Next, the witch sent the Winkies, whom she keeps enslaved, to do her bidding. They attack but are soon frightened away by the Lion's roar.

The Wicked Witch's final weapon is the winged monkeys. She has a magic cap that can only be used three times. It has already been used twice. She uses the cap for the third time to summon the monkeys. The winged monkeys grab the Tin Woodsman and drop him on jagged rocks, leaving him all battered and dented. The Scarecrow has had all his straw removed and his clothes have been left high up in a tree. The witch wants the Lion to be harnessed like a horse and puts him in a cage. This part is also simplified in the film.

The winged monkeys see the kiss mark on Dorothy's head and do not dare hurt her. They take her, still clutching Toto, back to the witch. The winged monkeys fly off, having kept their side of the bargain. The witch looks at Dorothy, with the kiss mark and silver slippers, and is afraid of her power; but she also sees her innocence, for Dorothy still does not know the power within her.

The Wicked Witch's weakness is that she cannot come into contact with water. She wants the silver slippers, but the only time Dorothy takes them off is when she washes. The Wicked Witch places an invisible iron bar on the floor, so that Dorothy trips and one slipper falls off, which the witch promptly grabs. Dorothy is so angry that she picks up a bucket of water and throws it at the witch, who immediately begins to

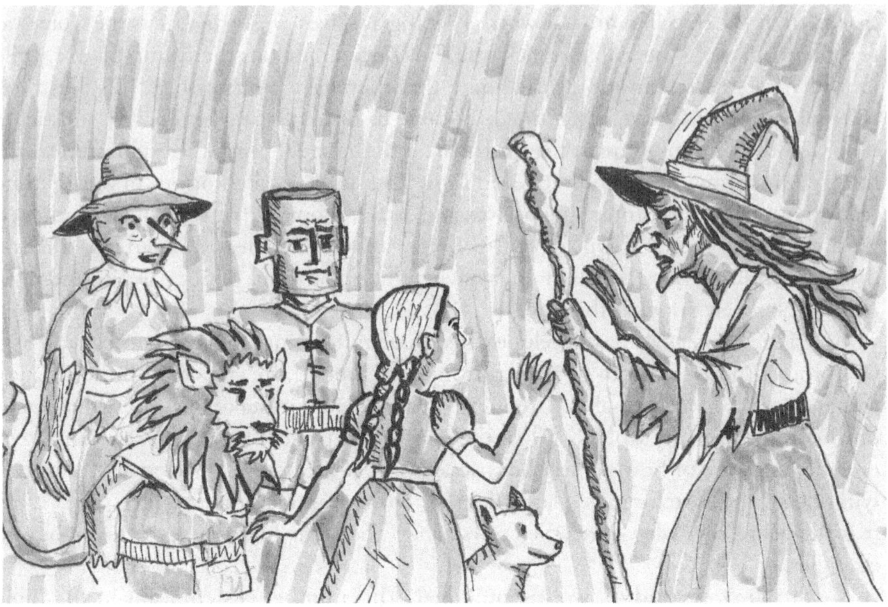

Figure 8.1 Dorothy and her companions confront the Wicked Witch of the West.

melt away. Once our shadow is seen to be what it truly is, with no substance, it must melt away. The witch's power lay in manipulating wisdom to conceal what was true. The film, again, is different. Dorothy and Toto get taken into the witch's castle, but Toto escapes. Meanwhile, the others manage to make their way into the castle. They get cornered by the witch, who tries to set the Scarecrow on fire. Dorothy then throws water on him to put the fire out, but the water splashes onto the witch, which causes her to melt.

Dorothy calls all the Winkies and tells them that they are free. The Winkies retrieve the Tin Woodsman from the rocks. Some of them were previously tinsmiths and are able to fix him. He needs some patches, just as our life experiences leave scars that need patching. The Lion is freed, and the Winkies find the Scarecrow and his clothes at the top of the tree. After recovering them, they bring the Scarecrow back to life. The Winkies give them gifts with many jewels to express their gratitude. When we have defeated our dragon, there is always a reward. Often, it is gold or the hand of a princess in marriage. We are no longer encumbered by those things that formerly held us back and we enter a richer life.

While Dorothy goes to get supplies for the journey back to the Emerald City, she comes across the Wicked Witch's magic cap. She does not know of its magic but chooses to wear it. This is another boon from having defeated the witch.

The group get lost on their journey back to the Emerald City and became discouraged. They call up the fieldmice, who tell Dorothy about the power of her cap and that the winged monkeys could take them to the city within an hour.

The Wizard

When they arrive at the city gate, they are allowed to enter again and word spreads that the Wicked Witch is dead. They soon find themselves in the presence of the Great Wizard. They can hear him but not see him. He seems to be delaying granting his promise. The Lion roars at the wizard out of frustration and startles Toto, who knocks over a screen. Behind the screen is a bald old man with a wrinkled face. He admits that he is the Wizard of Oz and that he uses tricks to make people think that he is mighty and powerful. He reveals himself as an ordinary person – as a fraud.

The sense of self – the ego that we have worked so hard to build over our lives – turns out to be a fraud. It seems strong and powerful, but it is ultimately revealed to be all too human. We create social institutions that seem real and powerful, but they are only as real as we believe. We came together as human communities and needed to align our ways of thinking in order to communicate, but it became all too easy to think that what we ended up choosing to believe was the actual truth. Each culture, each religion and each set of rules and laws tends to see itself as real, and to view whatever opposes or contradicts it as a threat.

The rule set is enshrined in the map, which becomes equated with identity. Any threat to identity tends to be perceived as existential and is therefore opposed and resisted. We do not usually change our map unless the cost exceeds the effort to retain it. The attachment to the social map is such that people are often willing to die for their country.

The sense of self constellates when we are young due to our life experiences. We absorb patterns from the people and society around us and imbue them with a reality that they do not deserve. We grow from being pre-conventional to conventional (Kohlberg, 1984), adopting the beliefs of the community around us. We are rewarded with acceptance by the community in which we live. We gain the support and approval of those around us, but at a cost. We have lost ourselves in our desire to be acceptable.

There will always be friction between what our society would like us to be and what we want to be. In some people, this dissonance is sufficiently weak to be dismissed; in others, it grows to become an overwhelming force. This heralds the shift to the post-conventional world. There is a cost when you break the conventional rules as to what is acceptable and what is not. Carl Jung said that we spend the first 40 years of our life building up our ego and the second 40 breaking it down again.

Thus, the curtain is torn away from the wizard and he is seen as the feeble, ineffectual old man that he is. Our individual identity is built on a network of metaphors that we have linked together in a way that supports our perceptions of ourselves and the world. As soon as we see the lie, we cannot unsee it and the whole edifice crumbles before our eyes.

Interestingly, we have defeated our dragon. This might seem to be a good place to end the heroic journey, but it is not the end. We must pick up the fragmented pieces of our worldview and start to pull them together in a new, more meaningful way.

Our whole society is built on lies. When we are young, we mostly absorb the values and beliefs in which we are immersed. We are told what is right and true; what is acceptable and what is not. We typically transition from pre-conventional to conventional, embracing the rules and constraints placed upon us by the society in which we live. We may live in a subculture, such as a particular religion or culture. As we grow and interact with the people within that culture – and especially if we have contact with other cultures and see different ways of acting – we start to see flaws in the map that our society has bequeathed us. Instead of being the one absolute truth, it is just one of many truths, and we start to envisage other ways of being. The wizard's trickery is built on lies; but if people do not recognise the lies, they give their power to the great liar, which feeds the great liar's ego to become even more extreme.

Buddhists believe that the self – who we are – is a fraud; a mere illusion that seems to be a particular way until we examine it closely. It is something that we have made up as we go along to enable us to cope in the world. The ego self becomes attached to seeking things that are pleasant and comfortable and avoiding anything painful or unpleasant. We are tricked into seeking physical gain, money, and influence. Over time – Buddhists would say lifetimes – we slowly come to realise that this is an endless search that can only bring misery. We must give up our search for fulfilment in the world of samsara, the world of appearances, for it has no eternal substance.

According to Buddhist teachings, we can transcend the world of samsara to reach a state of nirvana. The ego self cannot exist in nirvana. Nirvana is a state of being, not a place, as the Western concept of heaven is usually understood. It is beyond time and space. When experienced, it is a state of authentic, durable happiness. From this perspective, it is not so much about getting rid of the ego as such as about realising and releasing those illusory parts of the self.

When humans became self-conscious, we understood that death was the end of the self as we knew it – a terrifying reality to absorb and cope with, given that our whole purpose was to maintain and protect life. There will be a time when life ends. Ken Wilber (2007) suggests that this terror has been a powerful motivating force for us to create civilisations that will endure as attempts to break the ever-present threat of life ceasing. One could view a belief in an afterlife as mere wishful thinking to push away the existential fear of dying. The fear of death and how we resolve the terror it induces are part of our false self. This never goes away. No matter how strong our beliefs might be about life after death, we cannot definitively know either way until we actually die. Being at peace with the idea that I, as I know myself to be, will end, and that after physical death there may or may not be some form of ongoing existence, is a key part of the journey of transcending the false sense of self – the fraud that we perpetrate to maintain meaning in our lives.

Buddhist traditions embody ways of acting that lead us towards a realisation of the non-self. The self is attached to sensorial influences, so temptations such as money, power, greed, laziness, and aggression should be avoided because they all take us further away from realising the non-self.

Buddhists propose that meditation is the single best tool for coming to terms with the self and overcoming its intense control over our lives. Developing compassion and loving kindness is suggested to realise the oneness that we share with others and reshape the boundary between ourselves and others.

Note that the Buddhist use of the term 'ego' differs from the sense in which Freud uses the term. For Buddhists, the ego is the sense of self, bound by time and space, and tempted by all the things of this world, as mentioned above. Freud also used the term 'ego', but he saw this as the intermediary between the superego (the social mind) and the id (the emotional mind). After his enlightenment, the Buddha could still function in the world as a person. He still had an ego in the Freudian sense of the word but achieved selflessness.

When things go well for us, we tend to attribute this to our personality, skills, and abilities. When others succeed, we often attribute this to luck or other external factors. When we make a mistake, we tend to blame it on things outside ourselves, such as other people; but when others fail to do well, we tend to see this as a deficiency in them. In this way, we avoid having to look at ourselves and our mapping of ourselves and recognise a personal deficiency.

Gregg Henriques (2022) suggests that justification is a core driver of the ego. We need to maintain a consistent, justifiable place in the world that maintains our self-worth. He cites the example of a man in a bar who makes a pass at a woman. When she rejects him, rather than fully accept that part, at least, of the problem might be him, he will avoid the sense of humiliation by saying, 'She was interested, but she is just playing hard to get.' He has reframed what happened in a way that does not impinge on his sense of self-worth. Whatever our map shows, we will form a justification designed to enable us to continue using the map without changes, thereby avoiding the costly and energetic work of changing the map. A justification blocks out unacceptable ideas or concepts.

Abraham Maslow (1943) developed a hierarchy of human needs. The basic idea is that we start by focusing on our most basic physiological needs of food, water, and shelter. After that, we can focus on our safety and security needs. The next level up is love and belonging, which support the social aspect of our being; and then esteem, which is also a social aspect. We need an adequate level of status and recognition from the society to which we belong. At the top is self-actualisation, where we discover who we truly are.

Maslow's hierarchy was most famously illustrated as a pyramid, but in fact he never used the pyramid and probably would not have agreed with it. It makes the levels seem simple and logical, which they are not – and he knew it. All the levels are present at birth but they are not actualised until later. According to the pyramid, human connection is a need that only arises halfway up the scale. However, as we saw with babies sent to Romanian orphanages from the late 1960s onwards because of a national ban on contraceptives, a lack of connection immediately has a negative impact, rather than only becoming evident when they reach the next stage of development up the scale. While the babies had all their physical and safety needs met, their belonging and connecting needs went unsatisfied. They grew up to be severely underdeveloped.

The topmost layer in Maslow's model is self-actualisation. Self-actualised individuals are post-conventional and have their own voice. Unfortunately, Maslow was too much a product of his own society, which lauded the value of the individual over the community. I had a client who said, 'I have been told I must be self-actualised because I do not need other people.' Maslow self-selected people from within his cultural perspective as examples of self-actualised individuals, such as Albert Einstein, Eleanor Roosevelt, William James, and Albert Schweitzer.

However, people from other cultures – particularly Indigenous cultures – see such an individualistic perception of development as an error. The African concept of *Ubuntu* says, 'I am because we are'; while the Māori of New Zealand say, '*Ehara taku toa i te toa takitahi, engari he toa takitini*' ('I do not gain my strength from inside myself, but from being with my community').

The pyramid commonly associated with Maslow's hierarchy of needs suggests that no further development is possible once we have become self-actualised; but we do not know the limits to human development. Indeed, *The Wizard of Oz* suggests that once we have exposed the wizard as a fraud, much work remains to be done before the story is over.

We come to hear that the wizard arrived in the land of Oz by hot-air balloon as part of a circus. The balloon was caught up in strong winds and finally came down in Oz. While he presented himself as a wizard, he did not have the courage and wisdom to fulfil all that he could be. He ended up corrupting his power so that he appeared to be something that he was not and abusing that power to manipulate those around him, who treated him as a wizard and granted him their own power. While he did many things correctly, the impurities in his heart meant that he fell short of becoming what he could have been. Despite his weaknesses, Dorothy forgives the wizard for falling prey to the temptations that carry so many of us away. She does not become abusive or view herself as superior because she can see in her heart how she might have fallen herself.

The wizard tricked the people into wearing green glasses, so that they could only see their world in one way – the way the wizard had designed it for his own purposes. He was even able to trick the four witches of Oz into believing that he was powerful, so they avoided using their magic on him.

However, the wizard is able to tell the Scarecrow that he does indeed have a brain. The wizard creates a mixture and puts in the scarecrow's head, with pins sticking in it to indicate his sharp mind. It is not a brain; but it is enough for the Scarecrow to believe that it is, and he is happy. Next, the Tin Woodsman goes to the wizard to receive his heart. The wizard cuts a small hole in his chest and places a heart made of silk inside. The Cowardly Lion drinks a green potion to instil courage within himself. Toto's intuitive powers have always been intact and accessible. The journey along the Yellow Brick Road has brought the potential that sat within each of Dorothy's companions to life. Her own journey is now complete, as each of the parts within her has come together in harmony.

The wizard proposes building a hot-air balloon out of silk to take them away from Oz. He has grown tired of being a humbug and wants to fly away. He also knows that if the people realise that he is just an ordinary man, they will probably be angry with him. The wizard says that while he cannot be certain where they will land, they should surely be able to get to Kansas from there. It takes three days to make the balloon, and the Tin Woodsman chops wood and builds a great fire to create the hot air. Baum may have linked this three-day period to the three days of Jesus' crucifixion and resurrection. It marks the wizard's transformation from a false wizard to an ordinary person. This was not Dorothy's journey. For her to leave with the wizard would have meant remaining within the orbit of his illusion, still defined by the humbug, rather than discovering her own path home.

Everything is prepared and the balloon is filled with hot air, ready to go; but suddenly Dorothy cannot find Toto. Toto has gone into the crowd to bark at a kitten. By the time Dorothy retrieves him, the hot-air balloon has started ascending into the sky, leaving Dorothy and Toto behind. Once again, we see a mischievous, chaotic side of Toto that seems to be accidental; but this is actually the right thing to be doing. Had Dorothy climbed into the balloon, she would have remained stuck in the world of the fraudulent wizard. She would have been forever trapped at the conventional level, recreating the fraud wherever the balloon landed. The wise Scarecrow is left to rule the Emerald City in the wizard's wake.

The Journey to the South

The Scarecrow, the Tin Woodsman, and the Lion are all happy with how everything has turned out, but Dorothy still longs to return to Kansas. First, they summon the winged monkeys, but these creatures cannot travel beyond their land, so a wish is lost. They speak to a soldier, who tells them that Glinda, the Good Witch of the South, should know; but he warns them that a trip to the South would be very dangerous. Dorothy is determined to venture to the South nonetheless, and the Tin Woodsman and the Lion both decide to go with her. The Scarecrow also leaves with the group, promising to return to the Emerald City once Dorothy has made it home.

The group enter a dark forest. One of the trees reaches down and catches them, so they cannot move forward. The Tin Woodsman cuts off the branches and creates a pathway through. Again, there is another test before the next part of the journey can be undertaken.

Beyond the dark forest is a high wall made of china. The Tin Woodsman builds a ladder for them to climb over. Beyond, there are many buildings and even animals made of china. The people here wear white, gold, and purple – colours which are often associated with spirituality. China is fragile and can break easily. A cow made of china that a milkmaid is milking kicks over the milk bucket, breaking a leg off in the process. After deconstructing our sense of self, we are left in a brittle state and can break easily.

They next pass through a dark and boggy region, before arriving in an open area where all types of wild beasts are present. The Lion is addressed as the King of the Beasts. He is told that a large, spider-like monster has eaten all the other lions and is called on to defeat the monster. This is a test of his courage at the post-conventional level. He finds the spider, which is still sleeping. The Lion takes advantage of this, leaping up and taking off its head. The Lion says that as soon as Dorothy is safely back in Kansas, he will return to rule all the creatures in this land.

The next land that they reach is guarded by Hammer-Heads – strange creatures with no arms and flat heads that shoot forward and strike anyone who tries to pass. The Scarecrow and the Lion both attempt to get through but cannot. Realising that they have no other way forward, they decide to use their final wish and call on the winged monkeys. The monkeys carry them safely over the Hammer-Heads and into the land of the Quadlings, where everything is red. Once there, they are admitted to the castle of Glinda, the Good Witch of the South.

Glinda asks for the magic cap, which is now useless to Dorothy as it has already been used three times. Glinda uses the magic cap to send the Scarecrow back to rule the Emerald City, the Tin Woodsman back to rule over the Winkies, and the Lion back to rule over all the wild animals in the forest.

Glinda also reveals that if Dorothy simply taps her silver slippers together three times, she will be returned to Kansas. Had she done this earlier, however, she would not have developed as a person, as she has through her journey through Oz with her companions. Dorothy picks up Toto, taps her shoes together three times and suddenly finds herself back in Kansas with her Uncle Henry and Aunt Em, who have built a new house in the meantime. She discovers that her silver slippers have somehow fallen off on the way back home.

The final stage is always to return to the people from whom you came, to share the rewards and blessings of the journey with them. Jack returned from the beanstalk with a bag of gold, a goose that laid golden eggs, and a singing harp. Tāne, the god of the forest, came back from his journey to the heavens with three baskets of knowledge; and Jesus, resurrected from death, brought salvation to humanity.

In the book, we see Dorothy reunited with Aunty Em; while in the film, Dorothy wakes up to find out that her adventure was all a dream. She meets with the farmworkers again and talks about how there is no place like home.

In myths and fairytales, the good and evil characters are generally clearly distinct. We know who the goodies and baddies are. Gregory McGuire wrote the novel *Wicked*, which later became a musical and a film, adding a more nuanced extension to the original story. *Wicked* is written as an adult prequel to Baum's *The Wizard of Oz*. The Wicked Witch of the West, previously known as Elphaba, is depicted as being shunned because she was born green. This led to social exclusion and scapegoating. Glinda, previously known as Galinda, is depicted as a social climber who manipulates those around her to enhance her social reputation. In the prequel, Elphaba was a character of integrity, repulsed by the dominating control that the wizard exercised over the land of Oz. In contrast, the wizard and his power entranced Galinda. Further unfair treatment of Elphaba eventually prompts her to actively oppose the Wizard of Oz and Galinda, so she presents as an evil character when Dorothy arrives.

References

Baum, LF (2000). *The Wonderful Wizard of Oz: 100th Anniversary Edition.* HarperCollins and Wonderbooks.

Bocking, B (1997). *The Japanese Buddhist Worldview: A Study of Religious Philosophy, Symbolism and Ritual.* Routledge.

Campbell, J & Moyers, B (1988). *The Power of Myth.* Doubleday.

Henriques, G (2022). *A New Synthesis for Solving the Problem of Psychology: Addressing the Enlightenment Gap.* Palgrave Macmillan.

Kohlberg, L (1984). *The Psychology of Moral Development: The Nature and Validity of Moral Stages*. Harper & Row.
Maslow, A (1943). A Theory of Human Motivation. *Psychological Review*, *50*(13), 370–396.
Wilber, K (2007). *Up from Eden: A Transpersonal View of Human Evolution*. Quest Books.

9 Stories of Transformation

Introduction

We have explored the story of *The Wizard of Oz* in detail. Now, we expand on that with more stories. Myths and fairytales from around the world reveal the themes of the hero's journey and the principles of systems theory reflected in them. Each has its own approach and expresses the underlying dynamics in its own way, shedding light on the nature of archetypes.

The Crucifixion of Jesus Christ

The next tale that we will explore is that of the crucifixion of Jesus. The stories in the Gospels are factual recollections of historical events, but hidden within them is a far greater depth of mythological significance.

Myths have always been entwined with historical reality. Amazonian female warriors were considered fictitious until female warrior graves were discovered in the region. In New Zealand, the Māori had traditional stories of a giant eagle they called *pouākai* (or *poukai*), large enough to carry off a small child (Stack, 2016). *Pouākai* bones were eventually found. Homer's *Odyssey* was assumed to be a story until key geographic locations, such as the city of Troy, were unearthed (Jones, 2019). The tales of Jason and the Argonauts were similarly thought to be just stories about the golden fleece, until a place in Georgia was found where sheep's wool is traditionally placed in the river to trap gold coming downstream (Severin, 1990).

Often, a myth reveals depths that cannot be explained in a mere 'truthful' rendition of the facts. One example is the story of the temptation of Jesus in the desert by the devil. The Buddha endured a similar temptation. What would probably be seen by an objective observer in this story is Jesus going into the desert and finding a place to meditate or pray. Forty days later, he stood up and walked away. In his meditation or prayer, his shadow – represented by the devil – arose within him. His spiritual struggle with himself was mythologised as an exchange with the devil, where he was tempted by worldly offerings to abandon his spiritual search and return to ordinary life. By transcending these shadow constellations of inner mental activity, Jesus could return to his people with a true gift of transcendence. By mythologising the content,

DOI: 10.4324/9781003675266-10

we understand what happened, which could never be conveyed by a mere objective assertion of observed facts.

Jesus used parables as simple stories that convey a more profound truth. The story of Jesus' crucifixion is, in itself, a parable about the transformative process. The story is also fractal in that it can be read as a parable about one person's journey, a group's journey, or even the whole of humanity. It can be read as a parable about one whole life or particular events in a person's life. Just as myth distils the essence of many stories shared around the fire in traditional societies, parables gradually constellate into highly concentrated fractal forms. In this way, simple stories can transcend generations and are passed down to children and grandchildren. If one generation does not perceive the deeper meaning, the stories are simple enough to endure until the keys are unlocked by succeeding generations.

The story of Jesus follows the path of the hero's journey. He is brought up as the son of a carpenter, but is destined for more. He crosses the threshold in the Judaean desert and challenges the Jewish priesthood, dies on the cross, and descends into hell before being resurrected, bringing the gift of salvation. Let us now examine the story of Jesus' crucifixion more closely as a myth – not as an untrue story, but as a narrative that reveals more depth than a mere recounting of events.

Jesus enters the city to loud acclamations. Those at the height of the conventional lifestyle are praised by those who are also conventional. His actions to this point seem to be in harmony with how everyday people see the world. Jesus appears to be congruent with their maps, so no dissonance is felt.

From there, Jesus goes straight to the temple and throws out the moneylenders. Suddenly, he is acting outside the people's expectations and beyond their reality mapping. He is questioned by the religious leaders, who try to catch him out, but Jesus always has an answer that they cannot challenge. Jesus is operating at a post-conventional level. He is seen as rebelling against the accepted way of acting. The person who moves into the post-conventional world has found their voice and will speak their truth. They will inevitably clash with conventional people.

Judas, one of the 12 disciples, has stolen money meant for the poor. He quietly goes to see the priests and proposes betraying Jesus for 30 pieces of silver. The last supper before this betrayal takes place in an upper room. This symbolises Jesus having risen up through the levels of the mind to embody pure spirituality. After supper, Jesus says that he will be betrayed by Peter three times before the cock crows in the morning.

Jesus later falls to the ground and says, 'Father, if you are willing, take this cup from me; yet not my will, but yours be done.'[1] This is a puzzling statement. Two explanations are generally given. First, it reveals the depth of pain that he will suffer on the cross, taking all the sins of the world upon him because he is both fully human and fully divine. If crucifixion is the only way, then Jesus is ready. The second suggests that he fears dying from physical suffering before reaching the cross.

Jesus tells those with him to remain alert during the night, but three times they fall asleep right at the critical time. They have not elevated themselves to the level of consciousness where they can function as needed. They fall short. Jesus is seized and taken before Caiaphas, the high priest. Jesus poses too great a challenge to the worldview of the priests. As foretold, Peter is asked three times whether he is part of the group of people with Jesus, and three times he denies it.

The Gospel of Mark tells the story of a young man dressed only in a linen cloth who is caught by Roman guards but manages to escape naked. This could be an image to heighten the disappearance of the disciples as Jesus is arrested; or it might be a reference to the purity of spirit that is revealed and returned to life after the linen cloth (usually used as a shroud) is left behind.

The Betrayal

Whenever we move from a lower level to a higher level of functioning, we inevitably face betrayal. Those we have left behind see us as betraying their rule set and value system. We feel betrayed because they do not understand us and try to pull us back. An alcoholic who has decided to abstain from alcohol breaks the old drinking rules that kept the group together. The remaining alcoholics are challenged because, somewhere within them, they know that the sober person is doing what they do not have the courage or wisdom to do. The thought is too terrifying and unacceptable. A justification is formed. The rebel is demonised and scapegoated. The sober alcoholic feels alone and attacked. They need new social supports to replace those which they have grown beyond.

The dragon, as that which we are unwilling to embrace as a part of ourselves, is often scapegoated. The scapegoat pays the cost that we are not willing to bear. A justification story is developed that clears our conscience for evil to arise. We become the very dragon that we despise. We scapegoat in our personal lives, but whole nations and peoples can be scapegoated.

The actions of Judas in betraying Jesus led to Jesus' crucifixion and, paradoxically, to his resurrection. The betrayal of Judas is interesting. He has been condemned throughout history for his actions. He repents straight after the betrayal. He returns the 30 pieces of silver; and yet, had that not happened, there would have been no death and resurrection. This reflects the way in which the serpent is cast as the evil one in the story of Adam and Eve. The serpent is not lying when he says that Adam and Eve will not die if they eat the fruit and will become aware of good and evil. Without the self-awareness that arose in human consciousness, we could only act without awareness of our actions. The dawn of self-awareness meant that we could reflect on what we did and judge what was right and true and what was bad and wrong. Only then did we become fully human.

Betrayal occurs every time that there is emergence – a shift to a higher level of functioning. The old cycle clings on to what it knows and what fits its internal mapping. What emerges is a threat. It is necessarily a time of hardship and suffering.

We must ask why God would choose to create a world in which people can disobey and then become upset when people disobey him; or perhaps something more subtle is happening. Was it God's plan all along to create a world with people who can disobey him because the journey that we must now take raises consciousness? If we are all connected and God dwells within us, then the betrayal also ends up lifting God up.

Perhaps God is all-powerful and all-knowing, but made a mistake; or perhaps God is not all-knowing and all-powerful.

Is this the journey that God needs to be complete? If we are in God and God is in us, we have a creative role in making the universe. God needs us as much as we need God, in a co-creative journey together.

Pilate – the Roman governor of Judaea presiding over Jesus' trial – questions Jesus. The Jewish leaders are intent on having Jesus killed. Pilate tries to suggest a well-known criminal called Barabbas as someone whom the crowd might choose to kill over Jesus, but the crowd is determined to choose Jesus. Barabbas has not challenged the crowd's cultural map as Jesus has, so they seek to eliminate the post-conventional map that highlights their shortcomings. Pilate can see that Jesus is innocent of the charges against him, but fears the political consequences of freeing Barabbas. He therefore ritually washes his hands to absolve himself from blame for killing Jesus.

Jesus is publicly mocked, assaulted, and taken off to be crucified. Jesus hangs between two thieves. This links to the two demons at the gate of Buddhist temples. The world of appearances is divided into binary logic: a right and a wrong, two extremes. We think that we can look at a situation and decide who is right and who is wrong. However, when we do this, we lose the greater complexity and the nuances at play. What has become known as 'Hegel's dialectic' (Mueller, 1958) refers to the proposal of a thesis, which is the original idea. When we propose a thesis, an antithesis will arise in response. Both will appear to make sense, but they will contradict each other. Hegel suggested that a synthesis is possible, where the two sides of the paradox are resolved.

The Buddha lived a life of luxury as a prince in his palace. He realised that this would never bring him peace and left the palace to live the life of an ascetic – precisely the opposite. He similarly found that this extreme alternative did not bring peace. The true path was the middle way between the extremes, resolving the two into something new – something emergent arose from the interactions of the two. This is the middle path of Buddhism.

Jesus suffers on the cross and utters the words, '*Eli, Eli, lama sabachthani?*' ('My God, my God, why have you forsaken me?') Theologians have puzzled over these words for many years. For Jesus to be fully divine and fully human, it can be argued that he needs to feel the full despair of his humanity before it can be transformed into something new. This echoes his appeal to God to take the cup from him.

Then Jesus dies. His death reverberates through nature. The curtain of the temple splits and the earth shakes, breaking apart great rocks. This theme reflects the archetypal journey into the underworld found in so many cultures worldwide.

For transformation to occur, there must be a death. Old ways must be left behind for new ways to emerge. Particularly given our aversion to changing our map, this death is perceived as pain and suffering and a time of loss. All too often, we must hit rock bottom and have no alternative before making the necessary changes; or at least, the gains from transformation must outweigh the losses of the present moment.

The Gospel of John includes the story of a Roman soldier spearing Jesus in the side. From that angle, it could well be that the spear went inside Jesus' body and pierced his heart, symbolising the point of transformation – a change of heart – into something new.

Jesus's dead body is placed in a new tomb in a garden, reminiscent of the Garden of Eden. Jesus thus enters the realm of death. We hear that he descends into hell for three days. This is a common motif and is linked to the three days when the moon disappears as it nears the new moon and its reappearance after the new moon. On the third day, he rises again from the dead. The sepulchre is guarded to ensure that the body is not stolen and used as a pretext to say Jesus has risen. An earthquake strikes. An angel comes and opens the tomb, telling the people that Jesus is alive in Galilee. They find Jesus there. The Gospel of Luke tells of Jesus meeting a group of women on the road to Emmaus. The women do not recognise him until he breaks bread with them. Jesus appears to the disciples again several times and Doubting Thomas puts his finger in the wound in Jesus' body before he ascends into the heavens.

Orpheus

This theme of the descent into the underworld, is repeated in many myths worldwide, further reinforcing the universality of the journey into the darkness. Orpheus is married to Eurydice, who dies from a snake bite. Orpheus resolves to descend to Hades to free her. This is the descent into our own darkness, where we must come to terms with ourselves. Orpheus was born of gods and has their protection. He also has a lyre whose music enchants anyone who hears it. He convinces Hades to allow him to bring Eurydice back to life. However, there is one condition: he must not look back as he exits the underworld. Orpheus is unable to hear Eurydice's footsteps as she follows him and, at the last moment, turns to look back and therefore loses Eurydice forever. This represents someone who has descended into darkness but has not become fully transformed, remaining trapped and unable to move forward. Izanagi and Izanami share a similar fate when Izanagi looks back while bringing Izanami back from the underworld. A common theme in myths is the error committed, such as Eve's biting of the apple or Achilles' heel not being touched by water.

Heracles descends into Hades as one of his 12 labours, assigned to him by Eurystheus. He is told to fetch the three-headed dog Cerberus, who dwells in Hades. In hell, Heracles meets Pluto, the Lord of Death, who allows him to take Cerberus with brute strength if he can. Heracles manages this task and brings Cerberus back to Eurystheus. Cerberus is later released to return to Hades. We are reminded of Dorothy having to return to the Emerald City with the witch's broom.

Osiris

In Egyptian mythology, Osiris is a good king with a jealous brother, Seth. We again find the opposition of good and order and evil and chaos. They are complementary, interconnected forces in the world. There are many versions of this story, but according to Plutarch's version, Seth tricks Osiris into entering a coffin, where he is trapped, so that Seth can rule the two kingdoms of Egypt with his sister and consort, Nephthys. Seth throws the coffin into the Nile River. It ends up encased in a tree in the city of Byblos, resonating with the tree in the Garden of Eden and the wooden cross of Jesus. There might be a link between the winding river and a serpent.

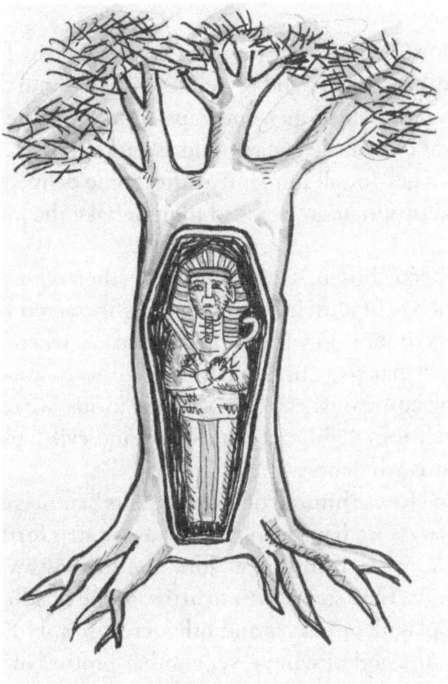

Figure 9.1 Osiris in his coffin encased in a tree in Byblos.

Seth then cuts the body of Osiris into pieces and scatters them over the land. Isis, Osiris's wife, gathers up the pieces and retrieves all of them except the penis, which has been eaten by a fish. She nevertheless uses magic to restore Osiris back to life. Osiris descends to become king of the underworld. Isis has a son, Horus, the heir, who eventually takes revenge for his father's death and reclaims the throne taken by Seth. Here, the theme of an old king and a new king arises.

Myths can be read fractally, so that the imagery holds for small events in our lives where we decide to do something differently through to an individual's whole life, and even through the journey of all humanity. When I first learned how to make a cup of coffee, I went through the same mythic pattern as when I met the most formidable challenge of my life. We see familiar themes and images repeated in cultures that were not in contact with each other. This points to deep psychological patterns that we share as human beings and that transcend culture.

Tāne Climbing the Heavens

Iain McGilchrist (2009) writes of the many myths in which two brothers are rivals. Drawing on the framework outlined in Chapter 3, McGilchrist suggests that myths of opposing brothers mirror the dynamic interplay between the brain's hemispheres.

The story of Osiris and Seth is one such example. The two are, in fact, complementary rather than opposing.

The traditions of New Zealand Māori[2] include the story of Tāne, god of the forests and of wisdom. He has a rival elder brother, Whiro, god of sickness, disease, and death.

Tāne and Whiro are sons of Ranginui, the sky father, and Papa-tū-ā-nuku, the earth mother. The supreme being decides that one of the gods should ascend the 12 heavens to receive the baskets of knowledge as a gift for all humanity. After some deliberation, it is agreed that Tāne is the god most appropriate to be asked to undertake the journey to receive the baskets.

Whiro thinks that he should have been chosen, since he is the firstborn. He grows angry and jealous. Here we have the image of a divine being in a highly sacred realm, beyond time and space, who sets events in motion within time and space, where dualities are present. Kant (1781) proposed that the mind creates the forms of time and space as the conditions for experiencing consciousness. Within these forms, we can see human experience unfold through dualities – light and dark, good and evil – playing out the eternal drama of moving towards wholeness.

Tāne undertakes purification rites to cleanse himself of impediments before crossing the threshold into the unknown realms. As we have seen, as soon as we step forth and take an action, we open the space for a reaction to that action. The shadow awakens and opposes that which has happened. As Tāne steps forth to arrive at the first heaven, he is followed by Whiro, who sends a plague of insects and other creatures. However, they are blown away by Tāwhirimātea, the god of wind – yet another brother of Tāne. This enables Tāne to step to the second heaven. Again, Whiro follows and attacks. This happens through all the heavens, right up to the eleventh heaven.

At the twelfth heaven, Toi-ō-ngā-rangi – the highest level of consciousness – Tāne can proceed, but Whiro is unable to ascend to this final level. Tāne has transcended duality and can enter the presence of the supreme being. Tāne receives rewards for his journey. He is given three baskets of knowledge: *te kete tuauri*, *te kete tuatea*, and *te kete aronui*. One version states that the first basket is filled with things that are helpful to mankind; the second is filled with the knowledge of sacred rituals; and the third is filled with evil knowledge. There are also stones called *whatukura* that hold the power of knowledge.

Tāne descends from the heavens to bring the gifts back to the people below. Whiro once more sends insects and creatures to attack Tāne, but they are again dispersed by the winds of Tāwhirimātea. Tāne comes back to the earth to share the gifts with all the people, as in the hero's journey.

Tāne is the god of the forest and of wisdom, linking the two concepts together. As we climb to higher levels of consciousness, wisdom grows. This links to the universal theme of the world tree. Odin hung on the world tree, Jesus hung on a wooden cross, and the Buddha found enlightenment under a tree. Jesus eats his final supper in an upper room to represent the ascent beyond the mundane world of everyday existence. A walking stick used at Māori gatherings, called a *tokotoko*, is a representation and reminder of the world tree, employed by orators in the ancient art of *whaikōrero*. '*Toko*' means 'to support' or 'to hold up'. A person is held up and supported in their search for wisdom. '*Whaikōrero*' can be translated as 'chasing words'. Standing in oratory, one must chase and find the appropriate words for the occasion. The *tokotoko* can also be seen as an umbilical cord, tying the person back to the land from which they were born and to which they will return on death. The world tree can further be understood as the human nervous system, starting in the roots and moving up into the brain and its more complex structures, where wisdom can be found.

Amaru

The Incas have a story about the twin-headed serpent, Amaru. The twin heads refer to the duality of the world. The serpent resides in the underworld of Ukhu Pacha. Amaru is revered as a guardian of wisdom and a symbol of water, fertility, and the cycles of life. During a time of drought and hardship, the unnamed hero is guided by the god Viracocha to approach Amaru. The hero must climb a sacred mountain, which is symbolically the same as the world tree. In doing so, he connects the underworld to the middle world and to the heavens. He must descend into the underworld, solve riddles, succeed at physical tasks, choose correctly in the face of moral dilemmas, and earn trust by revering the nature that is all around him. Having succeeded, the hero returns to the people with the knowledge of how to restore the cosmic balance so that harmony and prosperity can return.

The Kalpavriksha

Hindu mythology also has a version of the world tree – as do Jainism, Sikhism, and Buddhism. The Samudra Manthana is the churning of the milk ocean at the beginning of time. The *devas* (gods) and the *asuras* (demons) collaborate. Order and chaos intermingle such that life can spring forth. Out of this churning, the immortal nectar, Amrita, appears. As we move into the world of time and space, the world tree – the Kalpavriksha – emerges as a treasure in the world. It is a wish-fulfilling tree. The tree symbolises prosperity and abundance. Like other traditions, the tree serves as a link between the heavens and the earth. It is connected to the gods Shiva and Vishnu and the goddess Lakshmi.

There are further versions of the world tree in Viking lore, such as Yggdrasil, where the god Odin, wounded by his own spear, hangs for nine days and nights to retrieve the gift of the runes for humanity. The Mayans celebrated the ceiba tree, with roots into the underworld and leaves reaching to the heavens. In African mythology, the baobab is a tree of life. The baobab has a trunk up to 10 metres in diameter and can live for 6,000 years.

Māui-Tiktiki-a-Taranga

Māui is the youngest of five brothers and is a trickster (Reed, 2004). He resembles Loki in the Norse tradition and links to the jester archetype. He also has many adventures, tricking his way to success.

Māui is stillborn, so his mother, Taranga, wraps him in her hair and sets him floating on the ocean. Tangaroa, god of the seas, takes pity on him and keeps him safe. He is washed up on the shore and is found by his grandfather, who looks after him until he is fully grown. Here, we observe numerous connections between myths from around the world. Māui is again the outsider, the one who does not fit and who has an extraordinary birth. Osiris's body is put into a wooden coffin and set adrift. Perseus, whom we will read about soon, is also set adrift in the ocean. Moses is placed in a basket in the River Nile. It is like a sperm swimming through a great ocean to be fertilised into a new life and continue the chain of evolution from generation to generation.

Māui has many adventures, including rowing out to sea with his brothers in a canoe, which later becomes Te Waipounamu, the South Island of New Zealand. While out at sea, he raises the North Island of New Zealand from under the waves in the form of a great fish. Again, we see something unformed and hidden raised from the depths to emerge into consciousness. He steals fire from his grandmother, bringing it as a gift to humanity. Māui slows the sun, which has been travelling across the sky much more quickly. In the end, there is one challenge remaining to him.

Hine-tītama is the dawn maiden. She sleeps with the god Tāne, not knowing that he is her father. When she finds out, she decides to leave the world of light and descend into the underworld, remaining there as Hine-nui-te-pō.

Māui had heard that if he can pass through the body of Hine-nui-te-pō, death will be defeated and people will be able to come back to life, just as the moon returns after three days at the time of the new moon. Māui heads off with his companions, three small forest birds: a tatahore, a miromiro, and a tiwaiwaka.

Māui takes the form of a worm and enters the body of Hine-nui-te-pō. Again, we see a journey into darkness to overcome its power. The sight of Māui struggling to enter Hine-nui-te-pō looks very comical and makes the tiwaiwaka laugh. This wakes Hine-nui-te-pō, who realises what Māui is attempting to do. She crushes him to death inside her. Because Māui fails in his attempt to bring immortality to all human beings, we must die and return to the earth.

Yeh-Shen

Versions of the tale of Cinderella can be found all around the world. The story of Yeh-Shen was first published in the ninth century (Louie, 1982). Yeh-Shen has a wicked stepmother and an ugly stepsister. In this story, the magical wise person – the fairy godmother – becomes a magical fish. Yeh-Shen is the young, innocent hero who catches, feeds, and cares for the fish, but the wicked stepmother kills it.

A king hosts a grand festival for young men and women seeking potential suitors. Yeh-Shen attends but runs away before being recognised, losing a precious slipper. A villager finds it and presents it to the king. This is again one of those coincidental errors that brings enough chaos to change the direction of the story.

The king searches for the slipper's owner, but Yeh-Shen tries to take the slipper and is caught; it fits her perfectly. She leaves her stepfamily and marries the king, symbolising unity.

Don Quixote

The story of Don Quixote (de Cervantes & Smollett, 1605/2018) starts by describing the hero as deluded about his prowess and capabilities, as well as how he sees and makes sense of his world. This is, in fact, the state that we all live in. The world is not what we think it is. No matter how intelligent or capable we might appear, our knowing is always partial and we always misperceive the world that we live in. Don Quixote embodies the archetype of the innocent.

Don Quixote spends his time reading books, immersing himself in an imaginary world that is far more exciting and exotic. It becomes so real to him that he lives in this fantasy world rather than the real world. We live in the world of our making as we conceive it. Don Quixote sees himself as a bold knight and aligns his map of the world and the people in it to suit. He presents an unreal image of himself. He sees himself fighting dreadful dragons and defending the poor.

Of course, as he acts out this deluded sense of himself, the world keeps giving him information that shows how his map is wrong. However, he can always find a way to interpret the gap between his map and the world through another story, another justification. He is ridiculed by those who can see his folly; but actually, their lives are just as ridiculous. In his own way, Don Quixote is on a journey to go beyond his absurd and foolish ways of seeing the world. He is not satisfied with a simple, unexamined life, so he undertakes a journey that will provide him with the experiences necessary for a transformation into something new and more authentic.

Don Quixote makes a suit of armour out of bits and pieces that he finds about him and rides an old hack which, in his mind, is a fine horse called Rocinante. He leaves his house, crossing the threshold of ordinary life, and enters a new realm. Don Quixote finds himself at an inn that he believes is a castle and asks the innkeeper to knight him. The innkeeper goes along with Don Quixote's mad quest, but soon after, Don Quixote knocks out two guests at the inn who touch his armour and gets thrown out.

Don Quixote returns home, where he comes across Sancho Panza, a local farmer, who became his squire. Sancho is led on by the promise that he will become the governor of an isle and joins Don Quixote on his quest. Sancho can well see that Don Quixote is deluded and that he is no knight in shining armour. Yet there is a part of Sancho that recognises the spiritual journey he is being called to, and he also crosses the threshold to become part of Don Quixote's deluded vision. We can also see Sancho as an aspect of Don Quixote. He is the part still linked to sanity, mediating between Don Quixote in his madness and an external world in its own madness and delusions.

We gather people around us and weave them into our map, which becomes our reality. Rather than seeing people as they are, we see them as they fit into our mapping. Don Quixote forms the image of a woman called Dulcinea del Toboso and pledges himself to this lady.

Don Quixote and Sancho boldly go forth and fight monsters, which are actually just windmills. Of course, he cannot overcome the windmills. His lance is broken and he is knocked from his horse. We create monsters and demons in our fictitious world that we deem to be evil and must be defeated. It is so easy to label something as evil to

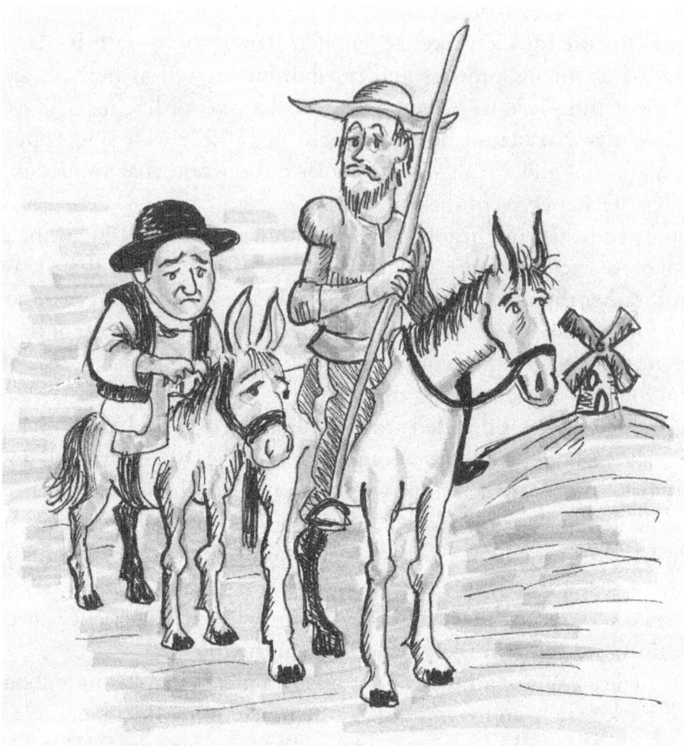

Figure 9.2 Don Quixote and Sancho Panza venture forth.

avoid facing that evil within ourselves. So often, the demons have no reality. The more we fight them, the more they create negative consequences in our lives.

Other people get dragged into Don Quixote's delusional world. Sancho goes up to a peasant girl and pretends that she is Dulcinea to try to end Don Quixote's delusion. A neighbour of Don Quixote, Sansón Carrasco, disguises himself as a knight to try to get him to return home. He has a shiny suit of armour, so is called the Knight of the Mirrors. Don Quixote becomes surrounded by people holding mirrors. He now sees himself as he really is. Finally, he reflects on his situation and realises that he is a feeble old man, not a gallant knight. We create a world of delusion; we call it the real world. Until we reflect on our situation and realise that the mental mapping we have created about ourselves and the world is but a fantasy, we cannot truly know ourselves. The knight's mask is removed to reveal Sansón Carrasco.

Now that Don Quixote has this insight, he must defeat the Knight of the Mirrors. On his way home, Don Quixote has several further adventures, including one where he bravely faces a lion that has been let out of its cage by a lion tamer. The lion shows no interest in Don Quixote and returns to its cage.

Don Quixote finally returns home. He is no longer a knight on an errand; he is merely an old man. He is also not the same man as he was before he became deluded. Just like Dorothy in *The Wizard of Oz*, Don Quixote went off into a fantastical delusion. He made his way through the illusion to return to the real world. From the outside, he seemed merely to be returning to how things were previously, but he has become a new man who has completed his journey and come home again as a whole man.

Notes

1 From Luke 24: 42–44, New International Version
2 Knowledge Basket, 'Knowledge Baskets Legend'.

References

de Cervantes, M & Smollett, T (2018). *Don Quixote*. Dover Publications.
Jones, B (2019). *The Discovery of Troy and its Lost History*. Trojan History Press.
Kant, I (1781/1787). *Critique of Pure Reason* (Transcendental Aesthetic, A22–A49 / B36–B73).
Louie, A (1982). *Yeh-Shen: A Cinderella Story from China*. Philomel Books.
McGilchrist, I (2009). *The Master and his Emissary: The Divided Brain and the Making of the Western World*. Yale University Press.
Mueller, GE (1958). The Hegel Legend of 'Thesis–Antithesis–Synthesis.' *Journal of the History of Ideas*, *19*(3), 411–414.
Reed, AH (2004). *Maori Myth and Legend*. Raupo Publishing.
Severin, T (1990). *The Jason Voyage: The Quest for the Golden Fleece* (New edition). Arrow Books.
Stack, C (2016). *South Island Maoris: A Sketch of Their History and Legendary Lore* (Classic Reprint). Forgotten Books.

10 Perseus and Andromeda

The Old Male Energy

This story from Greek mythology contains profound yet simply stated wisdom on the interactions of male and female energy. The hero of the story is Perseus, a young male, so the narrative describes the development of the male psyche as it grows towards wholeness. This version is taken from *The Greek Myths* by Robert Graves (2017).

Abas, the king of Argos, has two sons, Proetus and Acrisius. After Abas dies, the kingdom is left for the two sons to rule alternately. At the end of his term, Acrisius refuses to give up the throne. Bloody battles ensue and eventually the kingdom is divided into two. Here, we see the old male energy unwilling to give way to new, life-giving vitality. Acrisius has entered Holling and Gunderson's rigidity trap (2002) and desperately holds on to power through manipulation and violence; this no longer sustains himself as before, so it enters the release phase and breaks. What was once a vital and vibrant male energy has become rigid and inflexible. This rigidity makes it vulnerable and the inevitable pressure continues until the kingdom can no longer sustain itself; it then enters the release phase and splits into two.

Acrisius, now king of Argos, marries Aganippe and has a daughter, Danaë, but no son to succeed him. Acrisius visits an oracle to find out how he might have a male heir. To his surprise and anger, he is told that he will have no son but will die by the hand of a grandson. Other versions suggest that this is due to his quarrel with his brother. Acrisius represents the old male energy in the world, living by traditional patterns. He is told by an oracle – his inner wisdom – that his old patterns of expressing the male archetype will end, killed by a newer expression of maleness.

The old male energy is fearful of anything that threatens its perceived power. Its sole sense of identity is in its perceived power, so it will fight to the death to maintain control. It believes that by controlling people, it can maintain its position. The old male energy will commit any deed to hold on to power.

The king fights destiny to live beyond his time, leading a vampire-like, death-in-life existence. This blockage of the flow of life leads to him not having a son. Fearing the prophecy that his grandson will kill him, he attempts to control his outer world by arranging to have his daughter, Danaë, locked in a cell of bronze, guarded by two savage dogs. She must remain there until she can no longer have any children. In this

DOI: 10.4324/9781003675266-11

way, he seeks to avoid the birth of a grandchild, who might kill him, thus fulfilling the prophecy.

This is a typical response of the old male energy. It does not understand the female archetype and can only see it as a threat to be controlled. Acrisius thinks that he can lock his problem away; but we cannot lock things away forever in our unconscious world, just as the king could not keep Sleeping Beauty away from the spindle forever. Whatever is unnaturally controlled and suppressed will always find a way to reappear.

Zeus, father of the gods, comes down from Olympus in a shower of gold dust into Danaë's bronze cell and she bears him a son, whom she names Perseus. Zeus, being a god, represents inner wisdom, and this is an act of divine intervention that Acrisius cannot resist. Zeus brings new life and hope into a world of confinement and despair. We can compare this to a daughter who has been suppressed and controlled by her father. She reacts by rebelling and goes out to find a companion. She has not yet evolved enough for this encounter to become a full, long-lasting relationship, but the divine spark ignites a new understanding and perspective of the world. The encounter will be idealised; the companion will be made to be godlike. Danaë becomes pregnant. Danaë's encounter with Zeus is not simply a rape – if so, it would just be a continuation of her past oppression by Acrisius and would leave her without hope for the future. Zeus sees life from a broader perspective than Acrisius. Acrisius is bronze; Zeus is gold. Fight as we may, our inner wisdom will have its way sooner or later and will direct our lives for its fulfilment rather than our ego.

From this mixing of the divine male archetype with the female archetype comes the new male. New hope is born for males and females to come together. Significantly, Perseus's father is a god, which points to his greater destiny in integrating the male and female archetypes. Again, you will notice unusual birth events that mark out an extraordinary life.

As expected, Acrisius is furious when he hears of the birth. He reacts in the typical old male way of destruction and denial. Danaë and Perseus are put into a wooden chest that is thrown into the sea. In Acrisius's action, however, we see a hint of inner knowing within himself. Somewhere in his psyche, he knows that Perseus must grow to manhood, and that he himself must die. Acrisius could have had them both killed and ended the story there, but he chose not to. They are trapped in the chest – a prison, yet also a fertile womb. The chest is thrown into the sea just as a seed is planted into fertile soil to germinate. A spark of life is sent out through the unconscious world of the collective unconscious to float in the expanse of our minds. The chest is made of wood, an organic material from nature. It floats on the sea with divine help, a symbol of the unconscious mind from which conscious thought and action arise. Māui, the Māori demigod discussed in Chapter 9, was assumed dead at birth, wrapped in his mother's hair, and cast into the ocean, to be revived and cared for by his grandfather. We also see connections to the birth of Moses, the floating coffin of Osiris, and Noah's Ark.

In a way, the events thus far are a prelude to the rest of the story. The wooden chest represents our genetic, cultural, and spiritual heritage – those deeper parts of us that Carl Jung (1968) called the 'collective unconscious'. When we look deep inside, we find that we are joined to all other people. A part of our mind is shared with others.

Birth of the New Male Energy

The rebirth of Perseus on a new shore represents our own birth as an individual. A male child is brought into the world. Through his collective unconscious, he is already connected to and influenced by his past heritage. He will already have some inherent tendencies and predispositions, but his cognitive map is just beginning to take shape.

On another level, the events thus far could describe a marital breakdown, where the mother and child leave the chaos of marriage to a man of the old world and venture into a new world of uncertainty rather than remaining in a life-destroying relationship. At the beginning of the story, the female archetype is still undeveloped and lives in a 'victim' role until strength and insight allow her a more active role.

The wooden chest is washed up on the shores of the island of Seriphos. An island is a finite area of land within a greater ocean, which resonates with the idea of emergent behaviours arising as islands of order in a sea of chaos (Prigogine & Stenger, 1984). Indeed, birth is also an arrival into a place where life is limited. Emerging from the limitless collective unconscious, the soul enters a limited conscious life. These are enabling constraints (Juarrero, 2023) through which we can exercise power to act in the world.

Dictys, a friendly fisherman, finds the chest. He is a simple man who does not understand the complexities of life – just as it is for a newborn baby. He is also one who draws fish from the sea of chaos. This feels again like a wise divine protector, as it was for Māui, or even Jonah and the whale. Dictys, however, has a brother, Polydectes, who is the king of Seriphos. Polydectes represents the old male energy in our individual life – in contrast to Acrisius, who represents the old male energy in our collective life.

Perseus must learn new ways of being, which eventually means challenging the old energy. Here is the learning opportunity. How can Perseus transmute the old male energy if he does not meet, interact, and transform it in this earthly level of existence? Danaë and Perseus are taken into Polydectes' care and Perseus is brought up by him. (Although some versions suggest that it is Dictys who looks after them.)

Polydectes wants to marry Danaë. However, it is far too early for a marriage of male and female energy. The old male energy still has too much fear and denial, which would result in continued violence and abuse of power. Danaë's capacity for growth would die. The old king lives for lust, allowing his lower instincts to rule his being.

Perseus stands ready to defend his mother. He does not yet understand female energy, but he knows enough to realise that a marriage would be disastrous. He is also finding his own male power and using it correctly to oppose the king. For the old male, anything that threatens his power must be destroyed or controlled. He responds with anger and cunning. Lies, trickery, coercion, and deception are all deemed justifiable. We need only look at how easily we lie to ourselves to justify excessive use of alcohol, drugs, chocolates, or whatever vice we might have. We can always come up with a logical reason for our addiction. For example, we know that smoking is harmful to our health, but we might deny that smoking really is bad for us by saying, 'Just a few cigarettes are okay,' 'It helps me relax,' or 'I'll be lucky and I'll get away without health problems – my uncle did.'

Polydectes is also angry because he sees his own youth in Perseus. He once was an innocent youth with dreams and ideals of what his life could be like. He, too, once tried to stand up for what was right; but eventually he was worn away by the demands of the world and he conformed. How often do we see people with zest, vigour, and new ideas go out into the world, only to be worn down by the old ways of doing things, playing it safe? We must make mortgage payments and pay for a car, insurance, and school fees. Before we know it, all our old dreams have drifted away and we come to accept life as the same drudgery that we see all around us. All too often, we become part of the system that we once so vehemently opposed. Poor Polydectes, like Darth Vader, has been pushed down until there is nothing else to his life.

Polydectes pretends that he wants to marry Hippodameia, the daughter of King Oenomaus of Pisa, but in fact this is just a ruse to get Danaë for himself. Polydectes demands horses from all the islanders as gifts for Hippodameia. Horses represent our animal instincts. They are strong and powerful. Polydectes attempts to utilise his forceful, animalistic lower self to gain power over the female. He knows no other way to interact with female energy.

Descent into the Feminine

Perseus has no horses, so he is not led by his animal instincts; but since he sees that this is distracting Polydectes' attention away from his mother, he proposes a seemingly impossible and fatal task: procuring the head of the gorgon, Medusa. Different versions of the story suggest that it is Polydectes' idea to send Perseus to the gorgons, as he is sure that Perseus will not succeed. In taking on this task, Perseus has crossed the threshold. There is no turning back.

The gorgons are hideous old women with a seething mass of serpents instead of hair and tusks, whose mere look turns men to stone. The male energy is so trapped that it becomes totally immobilised and loses all vitality and life. Of the three gorgons, only Medusa is mortal, so it is she whom Perseus must kill. Medusa was once a very beautiful woman, living in a temple dedicated to Athena. Athena and Poseidon, god of the sea, had an argument, which prompted Poseidon to seduce Medusa to take revenge on Athena. Athena, in her rage, turned Medusa into a gorgon. We see here how a woman, or the female side of a man, begins with a natural beauty but, through mistreatment, jealousy, and envy, becomes embittered and hardened. She loses her beautiful shape and becomes hideous and unapproachable. We see the same vanity and envy in the story of Snow White.

The gorgons represent the old female archetype, worn and distorted. Perseus knows that his quest is achievable, even though he is aware that Polydectes sees no likelihood of his succeeding. Indeed, for Polydectes, there is no man who can approach the old female. All men who previously attempted this did so from within the framework of the old male and always succumbed to her powers, being turned to stone.

Perseus, however, is not afraid. Had he feared Medusa, he would have been defeated, as old energy lives off fear, not love. Fear is the dragon's lifeblood. The more we are afraid, the stronger the darker forces grow. The more we are filled with love, the less power the old archetypal energy has over us.

Perseus has committed himself to his adventure. He will never be the same again. At this point, as in so many myths and fairytales, a magical thing occurs. Athena hears all that has happened and comes to help him. She is partly motivated by her dislike of Medusa. At the point when Perseus is prepared to step forward into the unknown, the gods come to his aid. Once a commitment is made to growth and change in our lives, we contact the wise person within, who provides us with special insights and resources that we would not usually have access to. We need these for our journey, just as Perseus needs them.

The goddess Athena is the protector of heroes. She also provides Odysseus with vital assistance during his wanderings. She tells Perseus where to go to start his quest. First, he is sent to the city of Deicterion, where images of the gorgons are kept. Thus, when the time comes, he will know which of the three gorgons is Medusa. Perseus is warned not to look at the gorgons directly, but only at their reflections. The hallmark of human capacity is the ability to reflect. When we merely act out what we have done before, we act out of habit and cannot learn; however, once we step back and gain a broader perspective on what is happening, we can learn. Once you examine yourself as if you were a separate person looking on, you will learn about yourself in new ways and grow and evolve. Instead of just being angry, you become aware of your anger and can choose to act otherwise.

Perseus is presented with a polished shield that acts as a mirror. Hermes helps Perseus by giving him an adamantine sickle with which to sever the head of the gorgon. Perseus needs even more tools to help him in his quest, so he is sent to find the Stygian nymphs, from whom he receives a pair of winged sandals, a magic sack in which he can store the severed head and a helmet of invisibility belonging to Hades. These divine gifts appear only when Perseus steps fully into his task. In our own lives, a higher self can offer us the inner tools that we need to accomplish what would otherwise be impossible.

Only the three Graeae know the whereabouts of the Stygian nymphs. The Graeae are old hags who are sisters to the gorgons and who live on their thrones at the foot of Mount Atlas (or, in other versions of the story, in a cave in Libya).

The Graeae have only one eye and one tooth between them. Their energy has withered away and they have lost almost all true perceptions of reality and almost all true speech (represented by the eye and tooth respectively). When Perseus arrives, they refuse to help him. This is a test. They feel old, worn out, and threatened. They really want to be healed, but they must test Perseus to see whether this manifestation of the male archetype is sufficiently well developed to carry out the task of healing. Would Perseus be like the others and react with violence or wimpishly accept their refusal; or would he successfully pass their test?

Perseus grabs the eye and tooth as they are being passed from one Graea to another. He realises the core of their problem: their lack of vision and insight. He threatens to throw the eye and tooth into the sea unless they help him. He acts strongly, utilising the male attribute of direct action without resorting to the old, violent ways. As he is neither coward nor tyrant, the Graeae grant him what he seeks. Perseus has had his first experience of female energy and has succeeded in understanding the lessons. Because he understands female energy better, he also understands himself more deeply. Just as

Gretel finds the jewels of the old witch after she has overcome her, Perseus earns the gifts due for succeeding in the first part of his adventure when he meets the Stygian nymphs.

After receiving his gifts, Perseus embarks on his journey, flying west in the direction of the setting sun – towards death, darkness, and decay. He arrives in the land of the Hyperboreans, where the gorgons live. There, he finds the petrified images of men and wild beasts. It is men, with their animal nature, who are drawn to and bewitched by the old female energy. They became rigid and turn to stone after looking at the gorgons. When under threat, old female energy can be critical, callous, manipulative, and fierce. If the male does not have sufficient strength and discernment, he will come under the female spell and respond with fear or anger. A male without courage will withdraw under the threat of a critical woman. He will become increasingly tense and withdrawn, hoping to stave off further criticism. To avoid the hurt, he will deny his life force, becoming increasingly tense until he turns to stone. Perseus, however, represents new male energy and has courage. He does not simply react: he steps back to see the bigger picture of why the gorgons acted as they did and responds thoughtfully. He also has wisdom and the help of his higher self. He knows not to look at them directly.

The serpents on the gorgons' heads hark back to ancient myths in which feminine power is linked to serpents. We see this in the story of Eve and the serpent, where feminine insight and serpentine transformation are intertwined; in Greek figures such as Echidna, the half-woman, half-serpent mother of monsters; and in Ladon, the great serpent that guards the Hesperides' garden of renewal. Beyond its frightening shape, the serpent has positive characteristics. It is a symbol of rebirth: when a snake sheds its skin, it appears as a new creature. Within it is new life and regeneration, just as we see in the female symbol of the moon, which dies and is reborn each month, and in the female's ability to give birth. This female vitality must be released from its outer, frightening form.

We note that there are three sisters: three Graeae and three gorgons. The motif of three sisters is a common theme, as exemplified in paintings by Edvard Munch. The first is the virgin. She is the new moon growing towards fullness; she is birth, the beginning of things. Next is the pregnant mother, the full moon, the reaping of the harvest, the fullness of life. The third is death, endings, and dissolution; the waning moon, the old crone, the lady of the night. Māori tradition tells of Hine-tītama, the dawn maiden, who becomes Hine-nui-te-pō after discovering that her partner Tāne is also her father.

The gorgons live deep within a cave. They are asleep when Perseus arrives. They are spiritually asleep. Perseus must enter the dark unknown of the symbolically female cave to meet the female energy. He uses his magical gift of the polished shield and does not fall under their spell. He retains his integrity in the face of manipulation. The manipulation of Medusa can be compelling. It may appear logical and trustworthy, but it is a deceptive trap that can lead to disaster. A dispassionate, objective approach is vital. Emotions are likely to lead you astray. A reflective distance must be maintained and action must be clear and definite.

Perseus uses his winged sandals to hover at a safe distance; by viewing Medusa in his reflective shield, he can sever her head with a single blow of his curved

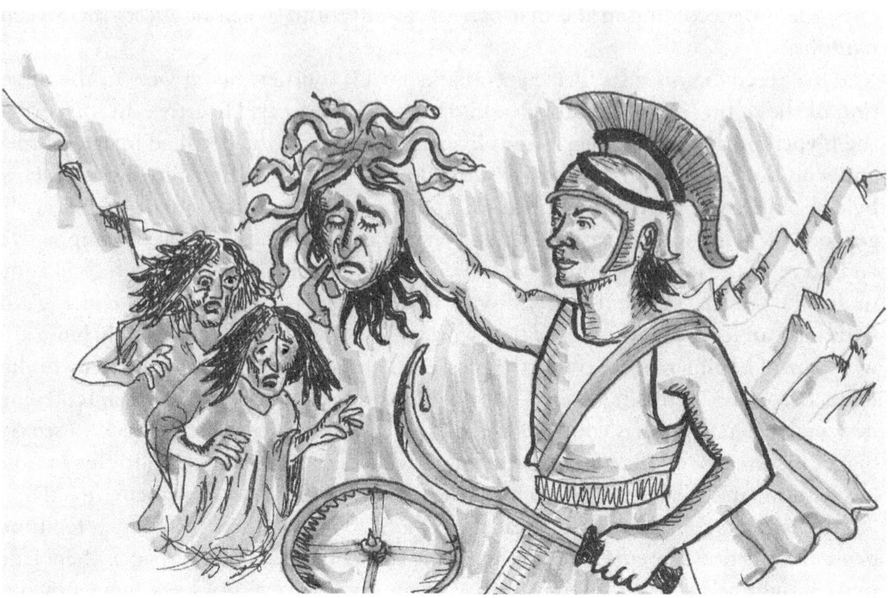

Figure 10.1 Perseus slays the gorgon.

adamantine sickle. This blow is struck with loving aggression. He is courageous and decisive, avoiding rage, revenge, or heartlessness. This is tough love. This is having the courage to do the difficult thing. This is better for the other partner in the long term. A partner in an abusive relationship who denies its abusiveness and never speaks up may keep the relationship alive in the short term, but they signal its death knell in the long term.

Eventually, the lack of courage will lead to the disintegration of the relationship. True courage is having the strength to stand up and risk a relationship, stating the truth as it is, so that true healing can take place. Had Perseus cut off the head without being balanced, he would merely have given the gorgons more strength. Heracles had to defeat the Lernaean Hydra, a seven-headed serpent. Whenever one head was severed, another two or more would arise in their place. Anger just grows and grows, becoming all-consuming. Hercules defeated the hydra by having his companion Iolaus cauterise the severed necks, so that they died, leaving Heracles the space to sever all heads. The hydra had one immortal head, which Heracles cut off using a golden sword given to him by Athena. When we see our emotions for what they are, they lose power. To face the old female energy with unbalanced rage returns our consciousness to our emotional self, which the old female is most adept at manipulating to continue the cycle of destructive behaviours.

As in the story of Don Quixote, a mirror is used to view a reflection. When we are consumed by anger, we are absorbed by it. We can learn to step back and reflect on our situation. While we are angry, we can learn to reconsider and objectively notice our behaviour and generate a more effective response.

Indeed, true healing arises from Perseus's deed. As Medusa's blood falls to the ground, Pegasus – the white winged horse – rises from her blood. Pegasus is a stallion, a male horse. The male aspect of Perseus is free to fly.

In her book *The Absent Father,* Alix Pirani (1989) suggests that there is no reason why we should not see Pegasus as androgynous rather than male. The horse can represent both male and female energy, set free. There is also a strong connection to free sexual energy and expression.

The shedding of blood within the cave of the gorgons is a symbol of menstruation. Blood is shed, but it is lifegiving blood. It flows with the rhythms of life and, if there is fertilisation, gives birth to a new creation conjoining male and female.

Perseus swiftly flies away using his winged sandals before Stheno and Euryale, the other two gorgons, can catch him. The newly born female energy is born. If the new male does not quickly move away, he will be caught in the backlash of the old female archetype.

At sunset, Perseus stops in the land of the Hesperides, where the titan Atlas lives. He is now beyond the human realm, as the newly found integration within him allows him to see new worlds that were previously beyond his gaze.

In a garden in the land of the Hesperides are the magic apples of Hera, wife of Zeus, guarded by Atlas, a great giant. You will recognise the similarities to the story of the Garden of Eden. In one version of the story of Heracles, he defeats a serpent called Ladon to retrieve the golden apples of the Hesperides. Perseus asks to rest in the garden overnight, but this is refused. During the argument and the struggle that ensues, Perseus draws the head of Medusa from his bag, turning Atlas into stone – Mount Atlas in Morocco, as we know it today. Perseus, with his new integrated self, has grown powerful. Atlas is male. He sees the true shape of the old female energy and evolves enough to incorporate the experience within himself, so he is turned to stone, just like the great multitudes before him. In one version of the story, Atlas, burdened with the task of eternally holding the earth on his shoulders, begs to look upon the gorgon's gaze so that he *can* be turned to stone and thus end his task.

The New Male and Female Energy

Perseus begins making his way back to Seriphos. However, it is too early for him to go straight there, as his newborn female energy – like any newborn – is still very vulnerable. Perseus flies to Chemmis in Egypt and Joppa in Philistia, on the coast of what is now Israel. Here, he spies a naked girl chained to a rock at the sea's edge. Her name is Andromeda. He immediately falls in love with her. She represents the new female energy. She is young, beautiful, innocent, and without shame.

She can show herself as she really is. Perseus can also see and accept her. Other suitors would withdraw at the sight of such nakedness. She is also naked because the experiences of this world have not yet clothed her. She is like a tender shoot struggling to grow and survive. This is a truly vulnerable time for her.

Her father, Cepheus, the king of Joppa, and his wife, Queen Cassiopeia, are standing on a cliff. Cassiopeia had vainly boasted that she and her daughter were prettier than the Nereids. The Nereids complained to Poseidon, who sent a flood and a female sea monster to ravage their coastline. This is the manifestation of the old energy, which sees the new as a threat and sets out to destroy it. The monster suddenly emerged from the sea, rearing up to wreak havoc and destruction.

After sacrifices prove unsuccessful, Cepheus consults an oracle on what to do. He is told that the monster will only leave them alone if Andromeda is sacrificed to it. If he does not sacrifice her, the monster will continue terrorising and devouring all the inhabitants of the land. Here, we see the negative backlash. The old energy wants things to remain the same. It pretends that things will be all right if they are like the old days again. This energy seeks to devour new life while it is still small, fragile, and vulnerable. It tries to use fear to stop the new growth before this becomes unstoppable. Perseus asks for and is offered the hand of Andromeda in marriage if he kills the sea monster.

Cepheus has not tried to stop his daughter from being killed. He thinks that he has no choice, since he is part of the negative complementary relationship with the old energy. The citizens call for Andromeda to die so that they might be saved. Every time the new energy rears its head, it is sacrificed for fear of its threat to the existing order of things. Cepheus bows to the pressure of his people and gives up his daughter.

Perseus is of the new male energy. He has true courage and wisdom. This monster must be faced up to before the new male and the new female can fully merge. If they tried to merge or marry at this point, they would be forced apart again by the old negative energy. Their relationship would break down. Andromeda would become the monster of the relationship. Perseus, therefore, goes forth, flying above the monster. Perseus is new energy and flying is something totally unexpected for the monster. The monster attacks Perseus's shadow, thrashing and writhing about in senseless rage. Then Perseus strikes at the beast with his sickle and cuts off its head. He has the gorgon's head to hand in case it is needed – and in fact, in some versions of the story, Perseus uses the gorgon's head to defeat the sea monster. Andromeda is safely returned to her parents, who are naturally overjoyed. Perseus makes offerings to the gods to give thanks for their help to him, just as it is right for us to be grateful for the higher energy we that we draw on to help us through difficulties.

Cepheus did not expect Perseus to succeed, so his promise of Andromeda's hand in marriage proves somewhat rash. Andromeda has already been promised as a wife to Phineas, a brother of Cepheus. Phineas is the male part of us that strives to gain the perfect prize before he has grown enough for a union to last. The rejection brings up feelings of jealousy. Phineas arrives with armed men to claim Andromeda. Perseus fights valiantly, but he is outnumbered by far. Perseus must thus use the head of Medusa to petrify all who seek to kill him.

Cepheus and Cassiopeia are set among the heavens as constellations. Cassiopeia, punished for her boastfulness, is placed on a celestial throne that turns upside down at certain times of the year. Cepheus, by contrast, is honoured with a stable constellation.

Perseus and Andromeda are married: the union of new male and new female. This is the mystic marriage of heaven and earth.

Perseus and Andromeda return to Seriphos. In the same way as a therapist takes us back to our childhood to re-examine our youth from an adult perspective, Perseus must return home. First, he must return to Seriphos and King Polydectes; then to Argos and King Acrisius.

Arriving on Seriphos, they find Polydectes still pursuing his mother, Danaë. She and Dictys are hiding in a temple. While Perseus and Andromeda were away having their adventures, Danaë and Dictys were back on Seriphos, undergoing their own learning. Danaë and Dictys enter a temple, a sacred space, for they too have brought their male and female energy together in a positive, nurturing way.

The old male energy of Polydectes knows nothing other than violence, lust, and greed. Any relationship that he might have would be based on those qualities and could never be fulfilling. Perseus leaves Danaë and Andromeda with Dictys and goes to the royal court to deliver his gift to the king. The gift, of course, is the head of Medusa. Perseus does precisely what Polydectes asked of him and shows him the head. As soon as the king sees the reality of the old female energy, his dancing partner, both he and those around him are filled with fear and turned to stone. These stones still stand on the island of Seriphos. Perseus puts Dictys on the throne of the island of Seriphos. A good king has finally arrived. Now sound wisdom and authority can spread throughout the island.

Hermes and Athena visit Perseus and he returns their gifts. Hermes will bring the cap, sandals, and bag back to the Stygian nymphs. Athena takes the head of Medusa, which she fixes onto her shield. We cannot remain in our higher self permanently. We cannot be forever meditating or having mystical experiences. Life is about learning to live on earth, with its restrictions. Now that the gods' gifts are no longer required, they are returned. The head of Medusa becomes part of Athena. The ability to stand up to the old female energy becomes part of our higher self.

Now it is time to return to Argos. Dictys remains on Seriphos, but Perseus, Andromeda, and Danaë travel on to Argos, where Perseus must face his destiny. He cannot rely on the gifts of the gods for his final task. In the end, we must take responsibility for our situations and face them as humans.

Acrisius still fears the old prophecy that he will die by the hand of a grandson. Unable to imagine forgiveness, he flees Argos and seeks refuge with King Teutamides of Larissa, who is hosting funeral games for his father. It is there, in this neutral setting, that the prophecy is fulfilled.

Perseus is invited to Larissa for funeral games that Teutamides is holding in honour of his dead father. As these are funeral games, we get a sense of the ending. This is the final challenge for Perseus: the last stand of the old male. Indeed, the old king archetype in this story is on the verge of death.

One of the competitions in the funeral games is the discus, reminiscent of the polished shield of Perseus. When Perseus throws the discus, it is guided by destiny and fate (some versions say by Zeus). It is picked up by the wind in mid-air. It veers off to the side, striking and killing Acrisius. The old prophecy is thus fulfilled. Although

Perseus has compassion for Acrisius and no thought of revenge, as the new male energy grows in strength, the old energy must die. Perseus cannot be the king ruling with new male energy while the old man lives. As Perseus grows in strength and spirit, Acrisius becomes weak. Perseus feels sad, but there can be no other outcome.

This is why Jesus tells the man who would follow him but wished first to bury his father that he must leave with him and let the dead bury the dead. Leave the old energy to itself. It is most likely that burying his father meant looking after him until he died. If any of the old energy is still alive as a shadow for Perseus, it will manifest later in his life.

Perseus buries his grandfather in the temple of Athena. Perseus is ashamed to return and rule in Argos, having killed the old king himself. He goes to Tiryns, where Proetus – brother of Acrisius – was once king. Proetus's son, Megapenthes, now rules. The two agree to exchange kingdoms and Perseus becomes the king of Tiryns. Now that he has found the new male energy within himself, he must make a fresh start. Had he just gone back to Argos to be king, he would probably have eventually turned into a king of the old energy; but by exchanging lands and making a fresh start, he ensures that his kingdom will remain strong. He will build great cities and rule wisely.

Perseus and Andromeda have children. Their daughter, Gorgophone, grows up with the new male and female energy around her. This gives her the strength to defy the age-old custom in male-based societies of the wife going to her death on the funeral pyre of her husband. The story is now complete.

At this point, it is worthwhile to look at the travels of Perseus throughout the story. We start on the land of Argos, on the Greek mainland. We then move south to the small island of Seriphos. From there, we move to Samos on the coast of Turkey and then make the long journey past Mount Atlas in Morocco to the land of the Hyperboreans, far to the north. Then Perseus returns to Africa, to Mount Atlas, across Libya to Chemmis in Egypt. From there, he heads to Joppa in Israel (although we also have a connection to Ethiopia through Cepheus). Perseus then returns home – from Samos back to Seriphos and then back to Argos. From there, he moves north to Larissa and ends up in his new home of Tiryns.

The shape of the land masses around the Mediterranean has been compared to the shape of the brain, with earlier civilisations springing up in the more 'primitive' regions of the brain. First, Perseus must go south, into the more primitive regions, to find his dragons, so that they can be healed. The location of the Hyperboreans' land is not definitively known, but because the word 'hyperborean' means 'far north' in Greek, it is assumed that the lands are located in the north. It would seem more logical for these to be further south, as it here that Perseus meets the gorgons – where he is in his 'darkest night'. Perseus returns via Egypt. The Bible uses the same imagery of travelling south into Egypt as a symbol of the descent into more primitive parts of the psyche. The Hebrew people are imprisoned in Egypt, from where Moses redeems them. On his return, Perseus has gone past the turning point in his adventure. He is gaining strength and power. He moves closer to home. As we explore our inner worlds, we go deeper into our unconscious selves. We go deeper into our childhood. Now that he has the key to his healing, he goes first to heal his male side at the personal level on Seriphos. Once the old male is transformed to that level, he descends further to the level of the collective unconscious on Argos and cures it. His final healing is even further north, in Larissa. With this healing complete, he can return to become king of Tiryns.

References

Graves, R (2017). *Greek Myths*. Penguin Books Ltd.

Gunderson, LH & Holling, CS (2002). *Panarchy: Understanding Transformations in Human and Natural Systems* (1st Edition). Island Press.

Juarrero, A (2023). *Context Changes Everything: How Constraints Create Coherence*. MIT Press.

Jung, CG (1968). *The Archetypes and the Collective Unconscious* (2nd Edition). Princeton University Press.

Pirani, A (1989). *The Absent Father: Crisis and Creativity: The Myth of Danae and Perseus in the Twentieth Century* (New Edition). Penguin.

Prigogine, I & Stenger, I (1984). *Order Out of Chaos*. New Science Library.

11 Eros and Psyche

Awakening and Separation

The Greek myth of Eros (Cupid in Roman mythology) and Psyche provides a balance to the more masculine hero's journey.[1] The story still has much in common with Joseph Campbell's hero's journey: there is the innocence that is broken, the descent into the underworld and the redemption and reward. However, while the male hero comes to know himself by acting in the world, Psyche learns by going inwards. There is a more receptive quality to how Psyche succeeds in the tasks that she is given. At first glance, it may appear that she is waiting for someone else to save her, but her receptivity is not passivity. She is turning inward, drawing on her deep connection to nature, and it is this inner alignment that allows the male and female aspects of the psyche to come together in union.

Aphrodite – the goddess of love, sexuality, and beauty – is the mother of Eros, who represents new male energy born of the eternal feminine. Psyche is the soul, the feminine energy, as yet innocent and naïve. Psyche is so beautiful that men are too in awe of her to approach her. Psyche grows lonely, yearning to become what she unconsciously feels within.

Psyche's beauty is so great that many consider her more beautiful than Aphrodite. This makes Aphrodite angry. Eros, her son, has a bow and arrow. Anyone struck by his arrow will fall in love with the next person they see. Aphrodite sends Eros to shoot an arrow at Psyche to make her fall in love with a vile, angry man. Here, we see the devouring shadow side of the great mother that must be overcome before we can come to know our true nature. We see a link between the overprotective mother and the coward discussed in Chapter 8. Out of her fear of losing him, the mother tries to control the son; but in the process, she hampers his growth. He must grow to become the warrior who meets his lover.

Psyche is the youngest and most beautiful of three daughters. Her beauty is so extraordinary that her reputation begins to eclipse that of Aphrodite herself, and this imbalance sets the curse in motion. Her sisters marry and have children, yet they remain unsettled by Psyche's radiance. Their jealousy is not merely personal; it is the shadow that rises whenever beauty threatens the established order.

DOI: 10.4324/9781003675266-12

Psyche's father, a king, seeks guidance from an oracle and is told that she must be taken to a cliff edge in mourning clothes. She is to be offered to a monster who will become her husband. This moment reveals the emotional cost of Aphrodite's curse. Psyche feels despair at her inability to find a partner, while her sisters embody the darker emotions that beauty provokes in others. Their envy is the human echo of the goddess's wounded pride.

You will notice the theme of the feminine waiting for the hero to come, rather than the hero venturing forth. Psyche is taken to the cliff as a sacrifice. The myth describes her as chained, but the chains signal her powerlessness rather than a literal restraint. A gentle breeze, the west wind, lifts her from the cliff and carries her to a lush valley with a hidden palace. There she meets Eros, though only in darkness, which preserves the pattern of the feminine receiving and enduring while the masculine remains unseen.

Eros is overwhelmed by Psyche's beauty and accidentally pricks himself with his own arrow. The gods possess eternal qualities such as beauty, wisdom, and love, but the challenge of life lies in how we apply these qualities in the real world and cope with the situations that arise from our interactions. Eros unconsciously realises that his pathway to self-development lies in manifesting the pure quality of love in his daily life. As long as the coward obeys his mother, she appears as the lifegiving, nurturing, caring mother; but when she perceives herself as being betrayed – as is inevitable – her wrathful, vengeful side becomes apparent.

Eros, too, has his shadow side. He is an adulterer and breaks up many couples through his mischievousness. Eros must grow out of his youthful, macho male behaviour to find the true meaning of love.

At this point, the relationship is unconscious. There is no complete awakening to the other. Psyche is more in love with the idea of love than with Eros. First love is often like this. Eros only comes to Psyche in the dark. She is not yet ready to see him as he is. He warns her not to try to see him, but that is just as impossible as God's expectation that Adam and Eve will happily remain forever in the Garden of Eden and never eat of the fruit of the tree of the knowledge of good and evil.

Even though their relationship is unconscious and in the dark, Psyche becomes pregnant. She longs for her sisters to come to see her and support her; but when they arrive, they are filled with envy, because Psyche has a divine partner – something that they can never access. As Psyche acts in the world, she creates a shadow. Envy and jealousy are often emotions that women tend to feel more intensely. Psyche has not yet developed the level of discernment that would allow her to see the error in how her sisters perceive her, and she is drawn into their mapping of the situation. Psyche feels her sisters' pull and they convince her to find out who her partner is.

Psyche is impelled to shine a light on Eros while he is asleep, to discover who he is. There is a link between the arrival of the sisters and the betrayal of Judas. This moment of seeing Eros in the light is also the same moment as Eve eating the apple in the Garden of Eden. When the unconscious becomes conscious, it is scary. It is the end of familiar things. Duality, pain, and suffering enter the world. Psyche brings a knife with her in case her lover turns out to be a dangerous monster. A knife cuts and divides things. When we shine a light on something, we see it openly and can separate and categorise. She drops the knife, recognising that Eros is not the monster that she expected. She realises that dividing and classifying the world is not the pathway.

Psyche is often connected to the image of a butterfly because of its metamorphosis from a caterpillar into a butterfly. This is an excellent representation of her journey towards wholeness. From a state of innocence, Psyche must individuate and find herself as a separate being; and once that is found, she must then integrate back with Eros in a whole new way.

Intimate partners cannot come together until they see each other in the light. In the dark, we can hide aspects of ourselves that we think will be unacceptable. In the light, these become obvious. We must learn to love our partners as they are, rather than the imaginary image that we might like to form in our minds.

In the light, the bow and arrow of Eros are revealed. Psyche is curious about the arrow and accidentally pricks herself, falling in love with Eros. Meanwhile, a drop of oil falls from Psyche's lamp and lands on Eros, waking him. He now also enters the light. Out of fear and a sense of betrayal, he regresses and takes flight. Each must then go on their individual journey of individuation, coming to know themselves, so that they can finally be reunited. The pair are now bound together in multi-layered, recursive interactions, including layers of suppressed emotion and trauma. They must find healing to reveal the possibility of discovering true love in the human realm.

Descent into Shadow

Psyche is devastated, thinking that she has lost Eros for disobeying his command. She enters the chaos and feels like committing suicide. She searches her shadow in a way that she has not done before and finds it frightening and overwhelming. She flings herself into a river, but it throws her back up onto the bank, where she is found by Pan, who advises her to return to Eros. Pan is the god of nature, reflecting the closeness of the soul and psyche to nature.

Psyche wanders aimlessly but eventually ends up visiting one of her sisters for comfort and support. She tells the story of how Eros abandoned her after she followed her sister's advice to look at him. Psyche decides to go to Eros. The sister leaves her husband to go to Eros; but of course, this sister, living in the shadow, can never be a partner for Eros. The sister leaps off a cliff, hoping the west wind will take her to Eros, but she falls to her death. The other sister does likewise. This is the outcome of living with such hurtful emotions.

Confronting the Wrathful Mother

Realising that the only way to find Eros is through divine intervention, Psyche is now ready to approach the wrathful Aphrodite. Aphrodite tears at Psyche's clothes and hair, asking her, 'What of your beauty now?' Psyche must have the strength to stand firm against the accusations of others. Many might ask, 'How dare she stand in the presence of Aphrodite, which so many others would never dream of doing?' However, like Arthur drawing the sword from the stone, she is the one who has the right to be there.

The Tasks of Individuation

As with the male hero, Psyche is tested. While this might appear to be an attempt by Aphrodite to stop Psyche by giving her impossible tasks, the tasks are exactly what she needs to individuate and know herself fully. Heracles is similarly given 12 tasks to complete. Psyche's first task is to sort all the grains in Aphrodite's warehouse. This is an enormous task that is well beyond any person. She must sift the wheat from the chaff. Again, Psyche must differentiate and separate before later recombining. Ants come to her aid and complete the task for her. Rather than the male action, Psyche is receptive, which brings the ants to her. You will notice that there is an intuition, a knowing, that comes to Psyche as to how she should approach each of the tasks given to her.

The next task is to retrieve wool from the golden fleeces of charging rams. The sun is high and very hot, which annoys the rams. The shining sun and the ram are masculine symbols. Psyche must find them in herself and not get swayed by the negative aspects. Water nymphs come to her and tell her how to safely complete the task: she should not attempt it at midday, when the rams are strongest, but should wait until evening, when their anger and rage have subsided. Then the golden wool can be retrieved from the trees that the rams brushed against as they charged by. Daoist philosophies and martial arts teach us not to engage our opponent directly, but to redirect the flow of energy to work in our favour, thereby defeating our opponent.

Psyche's next task is to collect a crystal flask of water from the River Styx, which is known to be poisonous, even to the gods. The eagle of Zeus – another symbol of male energy – comes to her aid, hovering overhead. Seeing her plight, the eagle swoops down to the river and fills her flask for her.

Psyche's final task, as in the hero's journey, is to descend into the underworld. She must collect an ointment from Queen Persephone. She again falls into despair. She sees a tower from which she could jump and kill herself. The tower is a masculine symbol, but she is not yet ready to engage in that journey. A tower is manmade and therefore relates to the level of culture. The allies that Psyche has received help from thus far have come forth from nature, but they cannot help her this time. Psyche must do this alone. Instead, she is advised by the tower (which can speak to her) to take coins for the boatman to cross the River Styx and honey cakes for Cerberus, the three-headed dog who guards the gates of Hades. She is also warned not to use any of Aphrodite's ointment.

There are further temptations that she is warned about that could divert her from her task, just as life presents obstacles that distract us from our true journey. These are reflections of the temptation of Jesus in the desert.

Death, Surrender, and Divine Union

Psyche almost succeeds but is tempted to look in Persephone's casket and take some of the ointment, so that she will look more beautiful for Eros. She falls into a deep sleep. This is actually the final release from her lower nature. Eros, divine love, awakens her. They are at last united in heaven. Eros takes Psyche to Mount Olympus, where she is accepted as a goddess and gives birth to a daughter named Pleasure (joy).

Note

1 This story can also be found in *The Greek Myths* by Robert Graves.

Reference

Graves, R (2017). *Greek Myths*. Penguin Books Ltd.

12 Jack and the Beanstalk and Rapunzel

Jack and the Beanstalk

Jack and the Beanstalk[1] is yet another story with much more depth than it is usually credited with. Noticing which characters are present and which are missing also gives us a clue about the intended audience. Jack has a mother but no father. His father has died, leaving Jack and his mother in poverty. This is the story of a young male growing up without a father – a scenario that is increasingly common today. Not having a husband has led Jack's mother to become bitter and resentful, which is evident in how she treats Jack and views her life.

Jack – a naïve young man – routinely forgets things, wanders off, does not complete tasks, and leaves burdens for his mother to bear. Their poverty, which in part has been due to Jack's carelessness, means that they must sell their one cow to survive. Jack is the innocent and incompetent youth who is still living the sheltered life of childhood.

Jack is sent into town to sell the cow and is instructed to get a good price so that they will have enough money to live on. Jack meets a funny old man, who convinces him to swap the cow for a bag of magic beans. In his innocence, Jack is tricked and returns home without the money that his mother is expecting. However, there is more happening here. The old man represents Jack's inner wisdom, which guides him on a path that will enable him to achieve far more. This is the same character as Obi-Wan Kenobi in *Star Wars*, Gandalf in *The Lord of the Rings*, and Toto in *The Wizard of Oz*, bringing wisdom to support and guide the young hero on his journey. Jack's mother, who represents the rigid and withered feminine energy in Jack's life, is angry at his stupidity. There are shades of the witch and the clown at this point. Jack's mother throws the beans out the window in a rage and they both go to bed without any supper. Jack's mother is still unconsciously alert enough to throw the beans where they will grow.

Jack wakes in the morning to find that the worthless beans have grown into a mighty beanstalk. He decides to climb the beanstalk to cross the threshold from innocence and undertake his spiritual journey of wholeness. The beanstalk is another version of the world tree discussed in the story of Tāne in Chapter 9. Jack leaves his mundane life behind and climbs forth into the world.

At the top of the beanstalk, Jack finds another world. He soon meets the giant's wife. She has a very different feminine energy from Jack's mother. She recognises that Jack is not yet ready to confront the giant and protects him by suggesting that he hide

DOI: 10.4324/9781003675266-13

in her oven, a feminine symbol of containment. Jack can witness the giant from the safety of the oven. The giant is none other than Jack's unresolved emotions, which have arisen from growing up without a father and with a mother who was unable to meet his needs. All his rage and anger, confusion, and resentment are embodied in the giant – a formidable opponent for him to encounter.

The giant arrives, shouting, 'Fee-fi-fo-fum, I smell the blood of an Englishman, be he alive or be he dead, I'll grind his bones to make my bread.' The giant's wife feeds him and he falls asleep. Jack manages to steal a bag of gold and returns with it to the bottom of the beanstalk. Fairytales often operate in a moral universe that doesn't map neatly onto real life, so Jack's theft is treated as cleverness rather than wrongdoing.

In the version of the story which Andrew Laing (2022) recounts in *The Red Fairy Book*, the giant killed Jack's father and stole all his gold. According to this version, Jack is reclaiming his birthright. This reflects how fathers are disempowered and taken away from their sons. The gifts and rewards have been stolen by the relentless patriarchy, which demands that men live in prescribed ways that alienate them from themselves and their sons.

The name 'Darth Vader' is commonly described as a variant of 'dark father'. The name 'Darth' was created by George Lucas as a variant of 'dark' and '*vader*' is Dutch for 'father'. While the name was invented before the decision was made that Darth Vader would be Luke's father, it is very fitting nonetheless. Darth Vader is a Jedi warrior who falls to the dark side. Our fathers so often give up their humanity and connection with their sons to meet the needs of a mechanistic, uncaring system that regiments and denies the human spirit. This is reflected in the way that Darth Vader is transformed into part man, part machine. So many sons grow up with a father who is absent, physically or emotionally. The pain of this separation becomes embodied in the shadow – whether that be Darth Vader or the giant Jack confronts.

Darth Vader sided with the Emperor Palpatine, using power and domination to achieve his goals, rather than love and connection. When Luke arrives as a burgeoning Jedi knight, Darth Vader must decide which side he will take. He could move fully into the darkness and kill his son; but instead, he chooses to return to Luke and find his humanity again. His mask is removed to reveal the man beneath. Father and son are reunited. Luke finds a new wholeness as his shadow is integrated. This leaves no space for the emperor to exist, because he represents the distance between Luke and his father, so Darth Vader throws the emperor into deep space. Darth Vader can now die because he is integrated; as can Obi-Wan Kenobi, as the trainer of Luke as a Jedi warrior. Obi-Wan Kenobi's death is actually a transformation into a new life at a higher level. His task is now complete.

At the top of the beanstalk, Jack has had his first glimpse of his shadow. He is not ready to see it fully. It would be overpowering and he would indeed be eaten by the giant. Very commonly, after confronting the shadow, there is a reward – which, for Jack, is the bag of gold. Jack has now moved from being pre-conventional to being conventional. He has money for himself and his mother to cope and survive. However, Jack's spiritual journey has only just begun.

Jack climbs up the beanstalk again and is again hidden in the oven by the giant's wife. He avoids the giant again but this time gets to see him. Jack becomes more aware of his shadow and its role in his life. Again, Jack receives a reward: he steals a goose that lays golden eggs and races back down the beanstalk before the giant sees him. This time, his reward is gold that will never run out, unlike the bag of gold. He is now very successful at the conventional level. However, he has not yet fully overcome his shadow – the giant still waits at the top of the beanstalk.

Jack climbs up the beanstalk again. Once more, he meets the giant's wife, who hides him in her oven. Jack sees the giant and steals his reward. This time it is a magical golden harp, which sings as music is played. This reward does not relate to possessions, as before. Jack has become post-conventional and has found his voice. He can see through the lies and errors of his conventional society. He dares to step forward and name what he sees. This links back to the different betrayals of the crucifixion: Jesus had to betray those who wanted to keep him quiet because he threatened their power base; while Jesus was betrayed by those who could not understand why he was breaking the conventional rules.

When the magical golden harp is stolen, it cries out, alerting the giant to the theft. Once we have found our voice, we cannot remain quiet when we see injustice. As soon as we speak out against injustice, we find ourselves to be the centre of attention. The

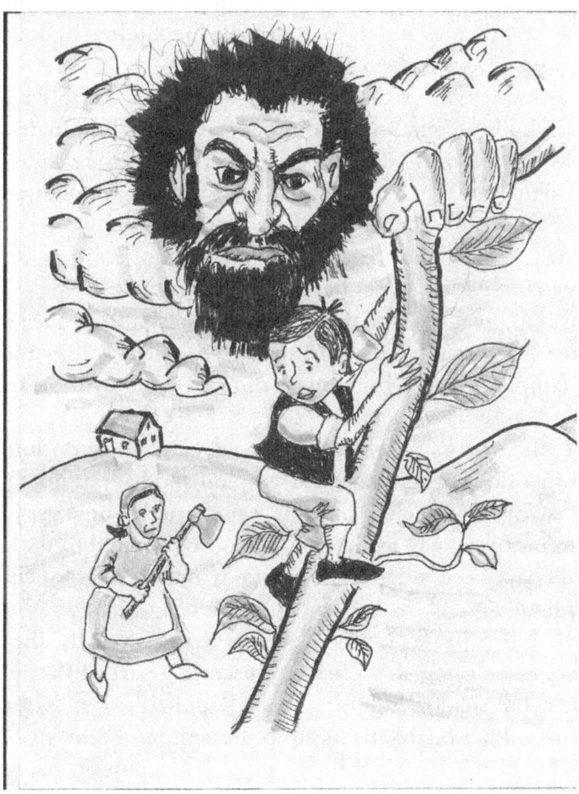

Figure 12.1 The giant chases Jack down the beanstalk.

shadow, fearing its death, strikes out with all its rage and venom. The giant chases Jack back down the beanstalk with the magical harp.

Jack's mother is waiting at the bottom of the beanstalk. She is no longer the bitter feminine energy, but is empowered and ready with an axe for Jack to cut down the beanstalk. The giant falls to his death. It might seem strange for Jack to cut down the beanstalk, given that it is the beanstalk that has enabled him to climb. Now, like Luke Skywalker, he has become whole. His shadow has become integrated. His male and female energies can now come together in a cosmic dance, where each co-creates the dance with the other. There is no further need for the beanstalk because the journey is over.

Jack and his family prosper with all the gold and rewards that Jack has found during his trips to the giant's kingdom. Jack has truly found himself in his post-conventional form.

Rapunzel

Next, we move to another story about women. The tale of Rapunzel is known from the Grimm Brothers' version, published in 1812 (Grimm & Grimm, 2023). They retold the story, which at the time would already have been hundreds of years old. They also reinterpreted it to reflect biblical themes and make it suitable for children in their eyes. It is therefore hard to know what was in the original story.

The story begins with a couple, who wish for a child but are unable to have one. As with all other fairytales, who is present and who is not is relevant. Both parents are present in the story, but – as we will soon see – they do not get to raise their child. They live in a small house overlooking the witch's garden. In her garden is rampion, a small edible herb, also known as 'rapunzel'. The woman feels an overwhelming urge to eat the rampion, to the point where she claims that she will die without it. There is a hint here that she is already pregnant, which causes her craving for rampion.

Her desire for the plant is so great that the man decides to steal it from the garden. This is the forbidden fruit that sets the story in motion. The man sneaks into the garden and gathers some rampion to take back but is caught by the witch as he tries to leave.

As with Adam and Eve, the man says that he only stole the plant to do his wife's bidding. The witch agrees that the man can take the rampion and have as much as he wants, as long as she can take care of the child once they are born. In some versions of the story, the parents try to move away to avoid having to give the child to the witch, but she finds them. It would have been much more common in those days for children to be brought up by other family members or even, as in this case, strangers.

There is a sense of inevitability. Just as it was inevitable that, eventually, the apple in the Garden of Eden would be eaten, it feels like a necessary part of the journey of growing up. Rather than the shadow resulting from Rapunzel's own action, the shadow is present by the time of her birth, arising from the actions of others.

Rapunzel is brought up by the witch. From the age of 12, when puberty begins, she is placed in a tower with no door. This is an obvious male image, where the male energy of the girl is stifled and unexpressed. There is no door to enter the tower, so Rapunzel remains entrapped by stilted male energy and the manipulative power of the witch in her female energy. Male energy is kept away from her because the witch knows that once Rapunzel realises her sexuality, she will lose her power over her. Without the evil overtones, there is a link to Miranda in Shakespeare's *The Tempest*, who is brought up on an island by her father and similarly knows no men other than her father.

The witch calls out to Rapunzel to let down her hair when she wants to visit her. Rapunzel's long hair is suggestive of both the flow of semen and an umbilical cord – links to the possibility of new life. Her hair is her link to her sexuality: it is beautiful and flowing, with promises of what is to come. However, right now, Rapunzel's sexuality has become rigid and trapped by the trauma of her past experiences and the events that have happened around her. The witch is named Gothel, meaning 'Godmother'. She tries to maintain her own sexuality by drawing on Rapunzel's energy through her hair, which the witch now controls.

One day, a young prince comes riding by. This is the new male energy, but it is still naïve and unrealised. He is naturally drawn to Rapunzel's beautiful singing, which he hears from far off while in the forest. At first, he goes away again because he cannot work out how to scale the tower wall; but his sense of enchantment is such that he is compelled to return to find a way to climb the wall. As the prince watches from behind a tree, the witch comes back and calls out, 'Rapunzel, Rapunzel, let down your hair.' Rapunzel lets her hair down and the witch climbs the tower. The prince sees this and learns how to reach Rapunzel.

The male energy is being called to the female and the old witch gives the prince the clue he needs. After the witch has gone, the prince comes forth and calls out, 'Rapunzel, Rapunzel, let down your hair.' Rapunzel does as she is bidden and the prince climbs the tower to behold Rapunzel.

Rapunzel had never seen a man before and is greatly puzzled and attracted to him. The two are entranced with each other and the prince asks her to marry him, to which she agrees; but she points out that the witch will not want this to happen and will try to kill him. The old feminine energy is threatened by the new, enlivened male energy and will try to destroy it to maintain its power. The prince leaves, promising to return the next day. The prince does not realise that the witch has been watching. The witch knew that this would happen one day, so she has always been on the alert.

The prince returns and brings a piece of silken rope each time, so that once it is long enough, they can descend from the tower and escape. A new link is being formed between the new male energy and the new female energy. One day, however, in her innocence, Rapunzel mentions to the witch that she is much slower climbing the tower than the prince.

Angry at Rapunzel, the witch climbs the tower and cuts off her long hair. When the prince returns the next day, he climbs the wall only to find the witch there instead. The old female energy has taken over and thwarted the growth of the new energy. The new male energy is full of hopes and dreams; but when the old trauma arises in a relationship, the dreamt-of relationship cannot sustain itself and the feminine energy lapses to the old feminine energy, destroying the relationship. In his grief, the prince throws himself from the tower, blinding himself on the thorns that grow around its base.

Now, realising that there is an imminent threat, the witch exiles Rapunzel to a far-off land, not knowing that she is already pregnant with twins. Despite all the witch's efforts, the sexual connection has been made and a new generation has been given birth.

The prince, in the meantime, wanders about searching for Rapunzel, and finally, one day, he hears her singing voice. He then comes across Rapunzel and her twins. It is a joyous occasion and Rapunzel's tears fall on the prince's eyes, healing him of his blindness. Love opens up a pathway for a healing transformation. The past trauma has been resolved and the two finally come together. They travel to the prince's land, where they live happily ever after. The male and female energies, after all that time, have finally come back into proper union in the relationship of the new sexuality that is lifegiving for all of them.

Note

1 This analysis is inspired by *The Sibling Society* by Robert Bly (1997).

References

Bly, R (1997). *The Sibling Society: An Impassioned Call for the Rediscovery of Adulthood* (Vintage Books Edition). Knopf Doubleday Publishing Group.

Grimm, J & Grimm, W (2023). *Grimms Fairy Tales* (1st Edition). Puffin Modern Classic.

Laing, A (2022). *The Red Fairy Book.* Independent Publisher.

13 The Homecoming

Introduction

We have now faced our dragons with courage. We have looked directly at what has been hidden and denied without turning away. We have looked deeply into our own hearts and owned what we found, no matter how uncomfortable that was. But we have not completed our journey. We still need to make the journey of homecoming. We must return from the fairy realms back into everyday life, to the people and places we started from.

The hero returns as a fully connected, whole person living in harmony with themselves and their world. The hero brings gifts – the results of learning gained on the journey – to be shared by everyone. Now that we understand the stories and their importance in shaping how we make sense of ourselves and the world that we live in, we can find ways to bring the archetypes alive within us to aid our healing journey.

We began by developing a framework for understanding ourselves and how and why we function as we do, particularly using a systems theory framework. The various models and theories are powerful tools that help us to make sense of the world that we perceive. We are now aware of many patterns in our everyday lives, which means that we can respond more effectively to the challenges that we face. If we can stand back from a situation, identify the dragon, and acknowledge it as a part of ourselves seeking healing, we can transform how we understand the people in our lives and generate alternative ways of acting to create better outcomes.

We will next cover some techniques that have been developed from this work that have been found to be effective. Note that they can be deceptively powerful. I conducted a workshop many years ago when I was starting out in this field, in which we visualised the core archetypes. People visualised seeing a representation of their dragon. For one participant, the dragon re-emerged while they were driving home and they had to pull over to the side of the road. I stopped running these workshops for several years. I now present this visualisation earlier in the day, so that help is available for people who might need it. I also carefully prepare people for the ways in which activated unconscious material may arise unexpectedly in a full debriefing session. I highly recommend that you have someone with you when undertaking this exercise, to support you should you need it.

DOI: 10.4324/9781003675266-14

Jungian Therapy

Therapies based on Jungian analytical psychology are a well-proven way of exploring and healing the psyche (Roesler & Reefschlager, 2022). Therapists are rigorously trained and have a wealth of experience helping clients to face themselves and encounter their dragons in a safe environment. Dream work is a key part of this process. The unconscious mind powers the dream world. The themes and images speak the language of the unconscious and are a doorway to discovering what the unconscious mind has to express.

Active imagination can also work. If we just let our imagination talk, it is surprising what we can reveal about ourselves. Word association is a technique where a client shares the first word that springs to mind when the analyst mentions specific words. Shadow work explores our fears and can help to bring forth the dragon in a safe environment.

Art and music are further tools. We can analyse a picture just as we analyse a story; images, colours, textures, and shapes will all have meaning. Sand play therapy is also used. All these techniques help to facilitate the process of individuation.

Meditations to Meet the Archetypes

Archetypes reside in our unconscious realms. There are times when aspects of our unconscious mind erupt and break through to our conscious mind, or when we can descend to meet them. The unconscious does not have access to language. Archetypes utilise myth and metaphor to convey their message. With an understanding of archetypes, we can translate these metaphors and hear the underlying message that we have kept from ourselves. We can create a guided visualisation to meet the various archetypes that we have come across, allowing them to constellate in ways that are meaningful for us.

Some people are very visually oriented and have no difficulty conjuring up complex and intricate archetypes, while others may find the archetypes presenting in different ways. There is no right or wrong way. Each person creates what they need.

I use one visualisation, which I have described below. Once people are guided into the house, a succession of archetypes can be met – as an example, I start with the king. The word 'king' will have different connotations for different people; other words – such as 'ruler', 'chief', or 'leader' – may evoke a more diverse range of images. You can then follow this with as many different archetypes as you wish.

> Get your body into a relaxed state and breathe slowly and deeply. As you feel yourself calm, close your eyes. Imagine yourself in a field in the countryside. Clouds skip across the sky; the warm sun shines down. Birds are singing and flying from tree to tree. There is the smell of country air and a gentle breeze that you feel on your skin. There are trees all around and a river flows past you to the side. You look to a corner of the field and see an opening with a gate. Notice what the gate looks like and how you feel as you pass through. You make your way to the gate and then walk through it. Follow the path through a garden that takes you to a house. Again,

notice what the house looks and feels like. The owner stands in front of the house as your guardian and bids you enter. Notice this person as you accept their offer and walk into the house.

You move forward and sit on a chair. The owner comes in to ensure that you remain totally safe the whole time. There is a knock on the door. Your first archetype awaits. You are perfectly safe. They come in. Notice how they look. Notice how you feel about them being in the room. They may be familiar to you or they may appear strange. There are no rules about how they should appear, but they do – they present a message.

Formulate a question for the archetype, and once you have spoken, sit and wait comfortably to feel an answer to your question arise. You may have another question or a comment for the archetype. Be open to the various ways in which a message might present itself to you. It may be a fleeting image, gone in an instant, an inner voice, or even just a feeling.

The archetype now gives you a gift in a box. Note what you observe in the box and give thanks for the special gift. The archetype will have a parting message that you may well find helpful. You can reply to the parting message and then bid them farewell as they leave through the door.

Next, invite the second archetype and repeat the process as many times as desired. After all the archetypes you wish to meet have come, bid farewell to the house owner and go back through the garden to the gate. Keep noticing everything that you see. Move through the gate back into the field. Notice what you are experiencing, but slowly bring your concentration back into your body and slowly bring yourself back into the room.

The dragon archetype is usually revealing and perhaps best left as one of the later archetypes in this visualisation. It is often uncomfortable, but it is the one from which we have the most to learn.

The gateway represents your pathway beyond the mundane world into a transformational space. The nature of the gate will reflect how you see your entry into that liminal space. The garden reflects the space that you move through on your journey; and the house represents you. They all send messages about yourself and your life journey.

Reflect on all the information that you gained about each archetype and the symbols that they presented to you. Notice who and what they were, their clothing, how they moved, the tone of their voice, the messages, the gifts, and more. They generally bring pertinent messages.

Dreams and Similar Techniques

Dreams are often a way for the unconscious mind to send us coded messages that can be unravelled. We do not understand sleep and dreaming very well, but this is undoubtedly a time to process unconscious material from the day and somehow put everything into context. Unconscious aspects of the mind often hold truths that we are unable or unwilling to hear, so courage is needed to peel back the layers and release the hidden messages containing the pearls of wisdom that we were looking for all along.

The hidden messages are conveyed through the use of metaphors and symbols in the dream. We can learn the code and release the messages and their meaning, helping us to gain greater insight into our internal processes. The unconscious mind can use language and puns. I once had a dream with a deer in it, which made perfect sense when the word 'dear' was substituted.

As well as dream content coming from the collective unconscious as a pool of shared images, we have a personal unconscious that holds events in our personal lives that we were unwilling or unable to manage when they happened. Care is needed because a dream can only be understood in its full context. Some books claim to interpret each symbol that arises in a dream. However, you can easily see how an obvious symbol might relate to a significant personal event for the dreamer with quite a different meaning.

We each have our own private store of metaphorical connections relating to our personal experience. There might be smells, sights, or sounds from our room as a baby, or the house we lived in, that trigger memories and connect in ways that others can rarely understand. I once noticed the smell of an apple as an adult, coming from nowhere, which took me right back to my mother giving me an apple in a park when I was very young.

We can practise and improve our ability to remember dreams. Some people find it useful to write down their dreams in a notebook as soon as they remember them. Merely setting an intention to be aware of dreams can help to build this skill. There are many books about the meaning of symbols in dreams. However, be cautious, because these books tend to overgeneralise and suggest specific meanings that might not be accurate for you.

Lucid dreaming is a type of dreaming where you are aware that you are in a dream and can consciously control what happens. In this state, you can do impossible things, such as walk through walls, fly in the air, meet people who have died, and ask for the answers to questions. Lucid dreaming can be a helpful tool, but of course, care is needed. If someone has mental health issues, it may be unwise; and some lucid dreaming techniques involve people waking up after a few hours' sleep, which – especially if repeated regularly – can lead to an ongoing lack of sleep.

While we are waking, there is an in-between space that we can enter where we are still connected to our unconscious but conscious enough to ask questions or direct the images that we experience. We can learn a great deal from this waking stage and learn to access it more effectively.

Beyond our dreams, we can access our unconscious in many ways. In everyday life, our mind is filled with the constant chatter of managing what is happening around us. Bruce Perry (Perry & Winfrey, 2021) distinguishes between the green brain, which manages the higher functions of thinking and social skills, and the red brain, which has the lower instinctual and emotional areas. 'Self-talk' refers to the constant voice that we hear in our head, which represents the conversation between the green brain and the red brain. When we chew things over, we tend to give the green brain time to present its perspective; and then the red brain gets a chance to make its case. Over time, we hope to balance out the two narratives into a single understanding that we can act upon.

We can choose to shut down the endless chatter, especially if it is too negative. When all that noise stops and we become alert to the more subtle movements and changes, we can hear a small, still voice that may manifest in a wide array of helpful ways.

In meditation, we relax and quieten our body, then our emotions, then our thoughts, and finally our social self. In that state, we are open to more nuanced influences that are more genuine reflections of who we are. There is a wide range of beneficial styles and techniques. Some use breathing because this unites our body with our emotions and cognitive processes. By focusing solely on the breath, we can better manage other distracting influences. Other techniques use mantras. These are words – often seen as sacred – that, if repeated over and over, can hold our minds from wandering and lead to flashes of insight and higher states of consciousness.

Relaxation techniques can produce a similar state of calm, openness, and receptivity. Visualisations are powerful ways of connecting with archetypes and parts of ourselves that need healing.

Journalling is another technique that can be done consciously; or alternatively, we can let our mind wander and write down whatever comes along. Some people find that writing with their non-dominant hand pulls the brain out of its habitual patterns and helps to access deeper content. Making a regular habit of journalling allows you to go back and recognise changes that might otherwise go unnoticed.

Movement can be used in the form of dance. Frenzied dance can help us to transcend our usual rational analysis and categorisation of the world, leading to greater insight. Movement in the form of tai chi or yoga can be powerful.

Dramatic devices such as psychodrama or family constellation work, where we take on the role of another person or even an archetype, can help us to connect more deeply. Therapy techniques such as Internal Family Systems (IFS) and psychoanalysis are also proven methods for accessing hidden unconscious parts and bringing them into healing.

Ritual is another technique that can help us to shift beyond our daily reality and connect with the divine within us. Ritual enacts psychic processes. In cleansing rituals, we might write down our thoughts or create something to symbolise an aspect of our life that we would like to leave behind. Having brought form to our fears, or whatever is the focus, we can burn, wash, or otherwise rid ourselves of whatever is causing us pain. Dance rituals evoke a sense of harmony in our bodies and create an atmosphere in which we feel safe to let go of unwanted emotions. Rituals can be individual or community based, where a whole group comes together for a special healing purpose. Drug-induced methods, such as rituals using psilocybin, have returned to popularity in recent years, with many claims of life-changing experiences (Goldsmith, 2010). However, these are often illegal and care must be taken with qualified supporting people to ensure your safety.

Storytelling

Dugyu and Yener Balan (2023) noted that cases of depression, anxiety, attention deficit hyperactivity disorder, and other psychological problems have become much more prominent in recent years. They particularly cite the COVID-19 pandemic; but other factors – such as climate change, unpredictable life events, social media, and an increased awareness of our psychological wellbeing – are also part of the mix. They developed storytelling techniques that plug into archetypes to explore new ways to address the myriad mental health issues that now seem to be appearing in our lives. They highlight the power of journalling by describing the emotions evoked by handwriting rather than typing on a keyboard. Writing with the left hand, which accesses the right brain, may bypass the left brain to access unconscious processes.

Backcasting

Backcasting (Inayatullah, 2022) is a process through which we decide how we would like our future to look and then plot out how to get there. The first step in backcasting is to understand where we are at present. To this end, we examine our cognitive map of ourselves and recognise ourselves, with all our strengths and weaknesses. The more accurately we can place ourselves, the easier it will be to navigate our lives using our map. If we are not where we think we are to start, we will get lost.

Next, we decide on a preferred destination or where we would like to find ourselves in the future. We live for the future. Our map should not merely represent the present or we will keep recreating our present situation and never move forward. Instead, we need to formulate a preferred future.

Having identified the two ends of the story, we can then backcast and fill in the events that need to happen to arrive at the preferred future. We end up with a plausible pathway from where we are to where we would like to be. We can apply the standard backcasting technique and turn the characters into fairytale characters. This is particularly powerful because the rational mind – which censors out anything that it feels might be threatening – overlooks the significance of the simple story and allows it to go into the unconscious, where its meaning is understood. This guiding story serves as a navigation star, drawing us ever closer to the desired future. Use your imagination to find suitable symbols and patterns of events that connect with the events of the backcasting. A group of people can collaborate on a story. I have conducted workshops where groups have devised stories around the various challenges facing humanity, such as climate change and international political instability.

During Donald Trump's first term as president, I wrote a story called *The Jester King* (MacGill, 2017). The story portrays Donald Trump as a jester who usurps the crown while the king is called away from the throne room. To his surprise, everybody takes him seriously and follows his commands, and he likes the role. A soothsayer comes and presents three potential future scenarios before the Jester King.

Write Your Life Story

The basic process of the backcast future can be used to gain a deeper understanding of ourselves by basing it on our own life story. We create a new story, redefining ourselves and reshaping our lives towards our preferred future. This acts as a dynamic blueprint of our future, drawing us in its direction.

I was born while my parents were on the verge of splitting up. As soon as possible after I was born, my mother returned to Nelson to her parents, but was unable to stay with them.

This was in the 1950s, and my sister and I were placed in the care of others. My sister was placed in an orphanage, while I was fostered by a family that I stayed with until adulthood. I took these events from my early life and mythologised them. A flying demon snatched me away from my family, leading to many adventures that culminated in me finding my long-lost parents and freeing an imprisoned princess. This technique implants a powerful preferred future that can reprogrammes your cognitive mapping towards your goal. For my story, see Appendix 2.

Causal Layered Analysis

Causal layered analysis (CLA) was developed to explore an issue by considering it on four interconnected levels (Inayatullah & Milojevic, 2015). Inayatullah uses the image of an iceberg because three of the four layers are not usually visible.

Only the litany level is visible above the surface. The litany is the first level at which we can see and understand a situation. A litany is part of a church service where a pre-set combination of words is recited together. There is no space to discuss the words or their meaning. The litany is the everyday level, where we take what we see for granted and do not look below the surface or explore any of the contradictions that might be apparent. Inayatullah uses the example of a newspaper headlines: you just see the bold, catchy title, with no content. We accept what we see without question.

Below this, however, is the systems layer, or the layer of social causes. Here, Inayatullah uses the word 'system' in a different way from how it is used throughout

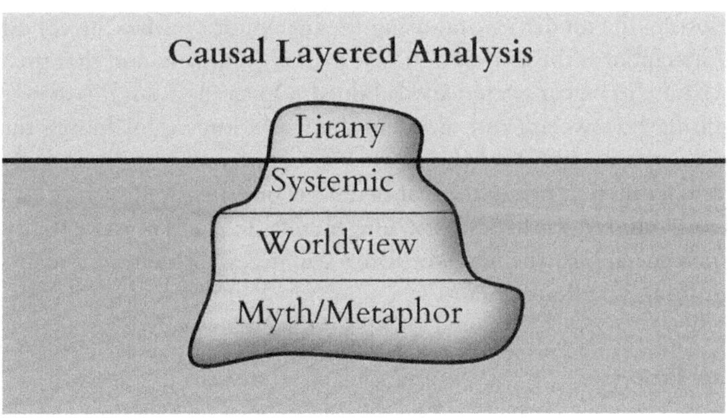

Figure 13.1 The CLA model.

In this model, the litany is above water and the system, worldview, and myth/metaphor layers are hidden beneath.

Source: Permission granted by Sohail Inayatullah.

the rest of this book. Inayatullah is describing a set of underlying societal rules and agreements that shape what a person can and cannot do at this level. Some rules are explicit and written into a code, while others are implicit. They are taught and become known as we grow up, so that we know how to behave appropriately in our culture. The economic, health, and education systems all function at the systems level to make the litany level possible. They tend to operate in ways that are invisible to the unobservant eye, yet our lives are determined by the rules that they impose.

Even deeper is the layer of the worldview. This is a consistent set of concepts and ideas that tells a coherent story about reality; about what is acceptable and what is not. The rules of the systems layer arise from the principles of the worldview. Truth is proclaimed at the level of worldview. It is not an eternal truth but rather a constructed truth that has become accepted and agreed upon over time. As long as people act as though the worldview is true, it has power – just as money has no absolute value in itself, but, because everybody agrees, pieces of paper or numbers on a screen grant access to services and resources.

Inayatullah proposes a final layer, which he calls the myth/metaphor layer. This means that metaphorical images, usually woven into a narrative, provide the core from which the worldview arises. The myth/metaphor arises from the unconscious, or is at least deeply embedded in the unconscious, and thus drives the way we act in the world.

You can see that each lower level feeds and shapes the one above. Donella Meadows (2008) notes that the deeper down we make a change, the more pervasive the outcome. I can only make changes at the litany level that are consistent with what is at the systemic level. If it is not consistent, I must make a change at the systemic level; however, I can only change something at the systemic level if it is consistent with the worldview level. Any changes at the myth/metaphor level can filter right up to the litany level. The deeper the level we are operating at, the harder it is to make a change, but the more powerful the changes we can make.

We might portray the modern world using the metaphor of 'Man the conqueror'. Hidden in this metaphor is the assumption that man is dominant, and that the world is something separate to be conquered and subdued. Operating from this assumption without recognising how we are embedded in the world leads to us killing the very environment that supports us. Our beliefs have consequences.

If we then find a different metaphor that better fits our situation, such as 'At home with Mother Earth', the old worldview is no longer consistent and must be reshaped to align with the new metaphor. The new worldview will necessitate a new systemic level, leading to a significantly different litany.

The Forgiveness Process

The forgiveness process[1] is a simple but powerful tool that we can use to free ourselves from the harmful effects of suppressed emotion. If we can identify someone who appears to be occupying the dragon position in our lives, forgiveness is a process of coming to terms with that person, allowing us to manage the suppressed emotions that were previously triggered in helpful ways rather than having them sabotage our

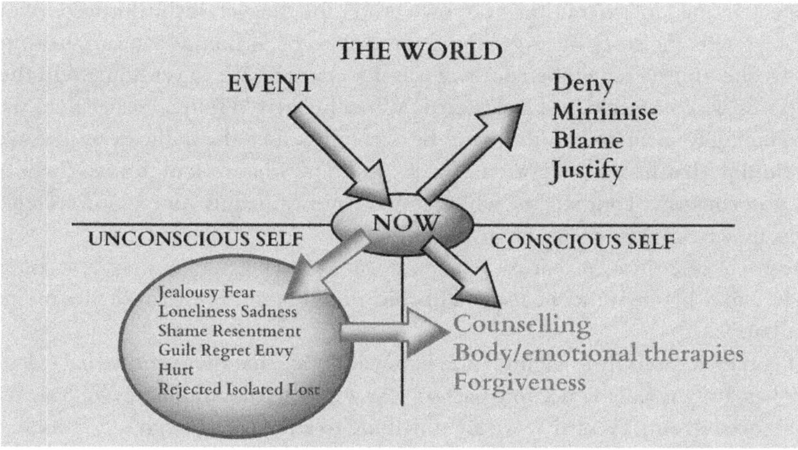

Figure 13.2 Healing suppressed emotions through forgiveness.

lives. It is an internal process and does not require the involvement of the person being forgiven.

The process whereby the emotions that accompany an event can enter the shadow are depicted in Figure 13.2.

We exist in the present moment at the living edge between us and the world that we live in. Events happen that enter the present moment. Some events are positive and align sufficiently closely with our existing cognitive mapping to become part of our conscious awareness. For whatever reason, there are other events that we are not as eager to make part of ourselves. We deflect these events and send them back out into the world. The event may be too intense for us to accommodate and would overwhelm us, so we cope by closing down. This is common in cases of trauma. The event may be too challenging for our cognitive mapping. It may be too difficult for our personal self-image. It may evoke uncomfortable emotions that we would rather not feel, such as shame and embarrassment. There could be a punishment or social rejection that would result. There are four ways in which we deflect events that we are unwilling or unable to manage in the moment. First, we can deny the event. We simply do not acknowledge it as real or valid. We often acknowledge part of an event to make it feel more manageable. The second is to minimise. Someone in a fight might try to minimise their actions as a push rather than a punch to avoid punishment. The third is to blame others. We avoid responsibility by attributing the cause of a misdeed to other people or to some other external cause. The person in the fight might protest that the other person started it.

Finally, we justify. We have seen this in Gregg Henriques' unified theory of knowledge (2024). To maintain a coherent sense of ourselves – especially when we have done something unwise – we often fabricate a justification that enables us to hold on to our old cognitive map and avoid the energy-expensive process of changing it.

It is only natural that we remember and recount events in our lives from our own perspective and tend to minimise our own errors and exaggerate the misdeeds of others.

Gregg tells the story of forgetting a promise to be at home by a certain time one day. By the time he remembered, there was not enough time to get home. On the way, the traffic was heavier than he expected. When he arrived home, rather than owning up to failing to meet his commitment, he overemphasised the traffic delay and avoided mentioning that he had forgotten. Once you know what to look for, you will notice how you construct your stories, which leaves you justified in your actions. Deflecting events may be conscious or unconscious.

You will often notice that two or more ways of deflecting events occur simultaneously. I may blame someone using a justification that minimises or denies my part in what happened.

If you look carefully at Figure 13.2, you will notice that the event we have deflected away has, in fact, already become part of who we are in that moment. We have already experienced it. Any event that we are unwilling to embrace through our conscious self must enter our unconscious self. This is particularly true for the emotions tied to the event. Feelings of hurt, resentment, anger, fear, loneliness, shame, guilt, frustration, rejection, resentment, and so much more constellate together in the unconscious to form the dragon.

If a person has had a traumatic experience, such as being in a car accident, future events that link in some way to the accident – whether that be going to the place where it happened or just hearing the music that was playing on the radio at the time of the accident again – can reactivate the emotions that arose during the accident. A threat response is triggered and often, while there is no rational reason for the emotions, they are experienced as real. Now, the person must cope with this new event and the recurrence of these old emotions. The old emotions do not arise cleanly, but as a dragon – they come forth in unhelpful and perhaps even violent ways.

If a previous partner cheated on you, your fears of abandonment tend to be heightened. You are looking for signs of a betrayal. Paradoxically, that suspicion can sabotage a perfectly good relationship.

Over time, suppressed emotions accumulate in our unconscious mind. We heal these emotions by bringing them across into the conscious mind. To shift them into the conscious mind, they need to be awakened and moved; the emotions must be reactivated and felt consciously. This is so uncomfortable that we would often rather let them languish in the unconscious. It is vital, when we wish to release suppressed emotions, that we do so in a safe and supportive environment in which we can cope with the feelings that arise.

A range of techniques can be used to help move suppressed emotions from the unconscious to the conscious mind. These include physical modalities such as massage; eye movement desensitisation and reprocessing – a technique that uses eye movements and has been found to be effective; holistic pulsing; and breathwork, to name just a few.

Expressing and naming our emotions can be beneficial. Writing them down in a journal can also be helpful. We can talk to a friend, a support group, or perhaps a counsellor of some type. Meditative practices such as tai chi and yoga, relaxation exercises, and affirmations can all help. Because we are fractal beings, any approach can provide a pathway to releasing emotion. We will find that specific approaches feel more comfortable and tend to work better for us.

As we move through old resentments, grief, anger, fear, and other emotions, we are less likely to be triggered by similar events that might arise in future and we can deal with those situations more competently. Carl Jung also wrote of the 'golden shadow' – those parts of ourselves that are so wonderful and amazing that we are unable to embrace them. We might fear that we will be unable to live up to the high standards that we have set for ourselves. We often have our hopes discouraged or even disparaged when we are young and are told to 'dumb down' so as not to be noticed. When the other emotions are loosened and freed, so is our golden shadow, releasing the full strength of our potential into our lives.

Our Full Bag of Tools

This has been a long journey of self-discovery. We have ventured forth through the enchanted land. We have faced our dragons and overcome them. We have gathered our gifts; and finally, we have returned home to everyday life. We are now complete and equipped to make better decisions about our future. We also have a toolkit of specific techniques to draw on as we work on ourselves to reach the point of leaving our safe haven, encountering our dragons and demons, and overcoming them. We have received our gifts and we are ready to move forward to heal ourselves and, through that, to heal others. We are back home among our people, but in a new way. We can be there for them and make a difference.

So, go boldly forth into the world, with all its challenges, using all the tools in your kit that will enable you to face your dragons and return to yourself and your community in a new way, invigorated and complete.

Note

1 This process is adapted from the work of Dr Guy Pettitt, who studied under Edith Staufer.

References

Balan, Y & Balan, Y (2023). *Re-write: A Trauma Workbook of Creative Writing and Recovery in Our New Normal* (1st Edition). Productivity Press.

Goldsmith, NM (2010). *Psychedelic Healing: The Promise of Entheogens for Psychotherapy and Spiritual Development* (Illustrated Edition). Healing Arts Press.

Henriques, G (2024). *UTOK: The Unified Theory of Knowledge*. Sky Meadow Press.

Inayatullah, S (2022). *Anticipation to Emancipation: Towards a Stage Theory of the Uses of the Future*. Https://Jfsdigital.Org/Wp-Content/Uploads/2022/02/Anticipation_to_Emancipation_Inayatullah-Final.Pdf.

Inayatullah, S & Milojevic, I (2015). *CLA 2.0: Transformative Research in Theory and Practice* (S Inayatullah & I Milojevic, eds). Tamkang University Press.

Meadows, DH (2008). *Thinking in Systems* (D Wright & C Labrie, eds). Chelsea Green Publishing Company.

Perry, B & Winfrey, O (2021). *What Happened to You: Conversations on Trauma, Resilience and Healing.* Flatiron Books.

Roesler, C & Reefschlager, GI (2022). Jungian Psychotherapy, Spirituality, and Synchronicity: Theory, Applications, and Evidence Base. *Psychotherapy, 59*(3), 339350.

Appendix I
Blimpo the Clown

One day, Blimpo the Clown was walking down the road when he came across beautiful flowers growing in the garden of Welda the Witch. He bent over to smell the flowers, but he slipped and fell, flattening them all. Welda the Witch came out of the house, screaming, 'How dare you do that to my flowers! Go away!'

'Oh dear,' thought Blimpo. 'What can I do? She is so angry at me. I know – I will do some of my tricks. Everyone likes my tricks and that will make her happy again.'

Blimpo picked up some stones from the pathway and started to juggle them, but one of the stones accidentally flew into the window of Welda the Witch's cottage, breaking the glass.

Welda screamed again, 'Get out of here before I turn you into a frog!'

'Oh no,' thought Blimpo. 'She is so angry with me. What can I do? I know – everyone likes my cartwheels. That will surely make her feel happy again.' He did a cartwheel, but he headed straight for her front door and smashed it into pieces.

'That's it!' shrieked Welda, promptly turning him into a frog.

Blimpo the Clown – now Blimpo the Frog – hopped down the hallway of Welda's house, knocking over a vase. A picture of Prince Ronaldo and Princess Alexia fell off the wall and broke into pieces.

'Get out of here before I turn you into a worm!' raged Welda.

Blimpo hopped out to the back garden behind Welda's cottage – and what do you think he found there? Thirty-seven other frogs, just like him! They told him that they had all done something to anger Welda and she had turned them all into frogs as punishment.

'But I don't want to be a frog for the rest of my life!' cried Blimpo. 'There must be something I can do?'

'Well,' explained the other frogs, 'We have heard that there is a witch called Briselmo who lives in an old cottage far off in the mountains over there to the west. She knows how to break the spell; but she is the most wicked witch in the whole world, and we are all too scared to go to her.'

Blimpo thought about this for a while and eventually said, 'I have decided I will go to Briselmo. I know she is terrifying, but I don't want to be a frog forever.'

Early the next morning, Blimpo gathered everything he needed for the journey and headed for the far-off mountains to the west. He hopped over the fence and down the

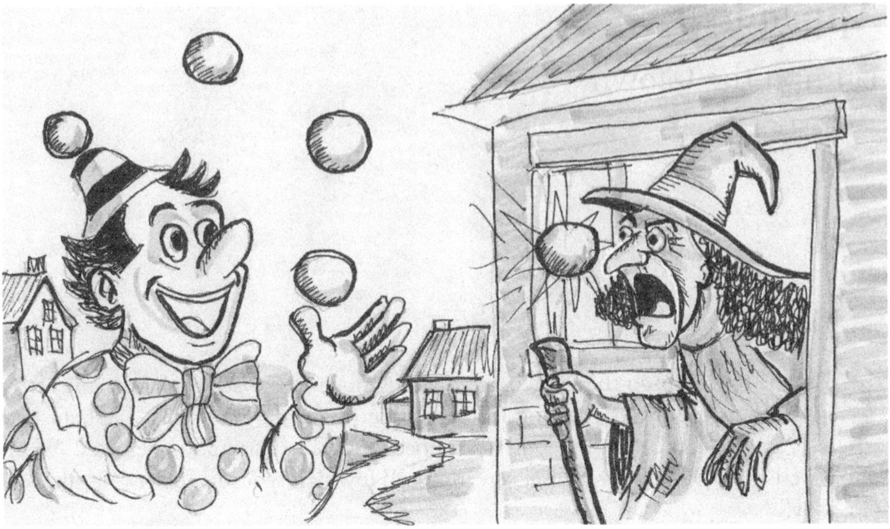

Figure A.1 Blimpo.

lane, travelled through the dark valley, crossed many rivers, and climbed mountains until he finally arrived at Briselmo's cottage.

He cautiously approached the door, took a deep breath, and knocked. At first, there was only silence, but then he could hear footsteps approaching. Briselmo, the most wicked witch in the whole world, was just behind the door. The door creaked open slowly until there she stood before him.

'Oh, how wonderful – a visitor!' she exclaimed. 'It has been so long since I had a visitor to my house. Everyone is so afraid of me that they never come. Do come in and have a cup of tea and some biscuits.'

Blimpo was rather taken aback by this friendly welcome but cautiously made his way inside and sat down while Briselmo made a cup of tea. As they chatted, he noticed a picture on the wall. It was the same picture of Prince Ronaldo and Princess Alexia that he had seen in Welda's house. He asked about it.

'Yes,' said Briselmo, 'they were the most wonderful people I have ever known. They were so happy, but one day I got angry and put a curse on them. It is the worst thing that I have ever done. I am so sad about that. But why have you come here?'

Blimpo told Briselmo all about the flowerbed, the broken window and door, and how he had been turned into a frog. 'I was told you could turn me back to how I was before.'

'Yes, indeed,' said Briselmo. 'What you must do is carefully go up to Welda, leap up, and kiss her on the cheek. But you must do this very carefully. If you make any mistakes, she will turn you into a worm and then there is nothing I can do.'

Blimpo finished his cup of tea and made his way back down the mountain, across the rivers, through the dark valley, down the lane, and over the fence. He told all the frogs about his adventures.

Soon, Welda the Witch came out to the back garden.

'Now is my chance,' thought Blimpo.

'We can't look …!' exclaimed the other frogs.

Blimpo hopped ever so carefully closer and closer to Welda the Witch; and when he was close enough, he jumped high into the air and gave her a big kiss on the cheek. Suddenly, Blimpo turned … not into Blimpo the Clown, but into Prince Ronaldo; while Welda turned into Princess Alexia! And all the other frogs turned back into the people they had once been.

Everyone was delighted to have Prince Ronaldo and Princess Alexia back among them. A big wedding was soon announced and Briselmo the Beautiful was the guest of honour.

Appendix II

My Story

On an island in a far-off land to the east, there lived a father and a mother. They were not rich but lived happily in their small, sunny valley.

The time had come for their child to be born. The mother gave birth to a beautiful boy-child. The mother worked hard to care for the baby. The father had been building a low brick wall behind their house before the child was born and soon after the birth, he returned to this task.

'I just need a few more bricks', he thought, picking up the wheelbarrow. As he started pushing it, he felt a shadow overhead, sending a shiver down his spine. He looked up and saw a black, winged demon circling high above.

As the demon flew down to attack the father, he threw bricks at it to drive it away. Though he fought bravely, he was no match for the demon, which swept down and struck him with its sharp claws. He was severely wounded and lay almost lifeless on the path, with a deep wound across his chest. The demon then grabbed the mother and boy-child and flew away high into the sky, leaving their fair valley far below.

The demon flew on for many hours over the sea until it finally came to another land. The demon was growing tired of the heavy weight of the mother and child. It could no longer fly as high and gradually dropped lower and lower until it was barely skimming the ground.

The mother looked down below them. There she saw a man and a woman on a beach. Taking her chance, the mother prised the boy-child carefully from the talons of the demon and dropped him the few centimetres to the ground. The demon felt the child fall and turned around, clawing at the child and wounding him on the chest. It then did the same to the mother. The man and the woman on the beach saw what was happening and rushed over to help, throwing stones at the demon. The demon left the boy-child behind but kept hold of the mother and flew off to the dark mountains in the west. The man and the woman picked up the child and took him home. They nursed his wounds, but he was left with a scar on his chest. They loved him and brought him up as one of their own.

When the boy grew into a young man, they told him how they had come to look after him. From then on, he dreamed of one day finding his mother and father. Eventually, he grew old enough to go and search for them. He bade a sad farewell to the man and woman who had cared for him and set out on his journey.

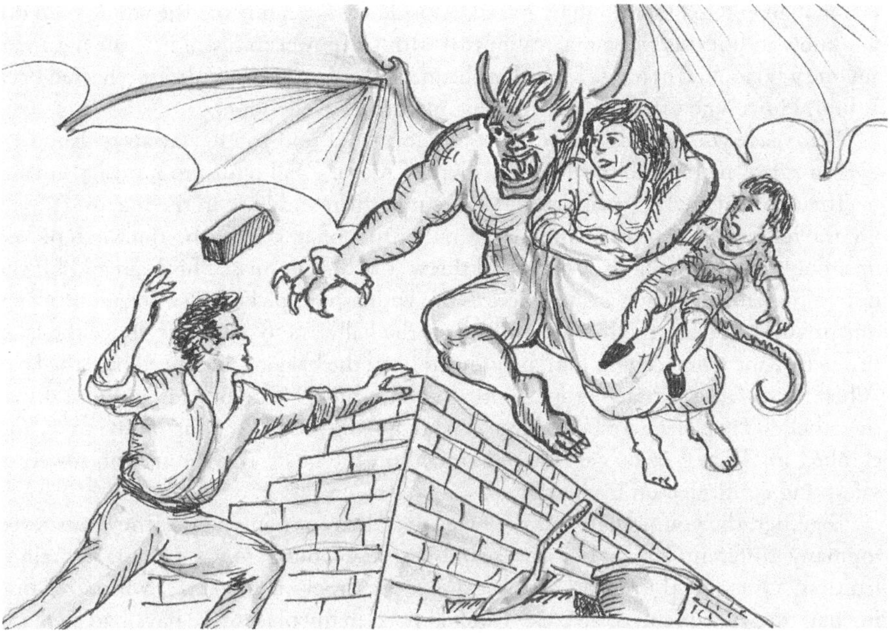

Figure A.2 My Story.

After several days, the young man met a strange old man, who was clutching a raven. He wore clothes the likes of which the young man had never seen before. He looked at once kind and gentle, stern and harsh. The young man wanted to rush on by, but was somehow fascinated by the old man.

'Well, young man,' said the old man. 'Where are you going?

'I am searching for my parents,' he replied.

'Ah – so where will you look?'

'I do not know,' admitted the young man. 'I have not been looking long.'

The old man then said, 'Give me your beautiful coat and I will give you this raven. It is a magical bird that will lead you to your parents.'

The young man thought about this offer for a while, because he liked his coat very much. He was also a little scared of the raven's stern look, but he wanted to find his parents so much that he willingly gave his coat to the old man.

The young man and the raven travelled until they reached a castle beside a lake. He was tired and weary. He knocked on the door and a gentle older woman answered. She invited him to stay the night and gave him food. She took him to a room where he could sleep. The woman told him there was one room next to his in the castle that he must not enter.

Later that night, the young man decided to look around the castle. He went and explored the different rooms and gazed out over the lake. It was dark when he returned to his quarters. However, the raven was waiting outside the forbidden room, so the young man entered that room by mistake. Inside, he saw a mirror. The young man did not know it, but this was a magical mirror with the power to reveal the true nature of anyone who looked in it. He looked in the mirror and saw his pure heart reflected back at him. However, at that moment, the woman entered the room.

'Why have you entered this room?' she shouted. 'I told you to stay away from it!'

'I'm sorry,' he replied. 'I came to the wrong room. I will return to mine.'

The raven squawked, making the young man turn and look in the mirror. He saw not the reflection of the old woman, but rather that of an evil witch. The witch picked up a book which was close at hand and threw it at him; it missed his head and hit the mirror instead, smashing it into pieces. The young man picked up a fragment of the mirror and fled from the room and through the hallways to a balcony above the lake. Just before the witch caught him, he jumped from the balcony and dived into the lake. When he surfaced, he saw a rope floating next to him. He grabbed it and found that the other end was tied to a boat. He swam across to the boat, pulling on the rope, and climbed in. The raven flew down and landed on the boat. The young man rowed to safety and continued on his journey.

Together, the young man and the raven travelled for many years. They journeyed to many different lands, but the search for the young man's parents remained fruitless. One day, the young man sat down on a rock in despair. 'I will never find my parents,' he lamented. 'We have looked in so many places. We have had so many adventures, but we've found no trace of them.' Exhausted, he sank to the floor and fell asleep.

When the young man woke, he saw an old man looking down at him.

'Young man, why are you sleeping out here where it is so cold?'

The young man sat up and replied, 'I am on a quest to find my parents. I have searched so many lands and places, but I have found no trace of them. I was given this magic raven to help me, but still I have found no trace of them. I am so weary from my travels.'

With that, he slumped to the ground again. As he did, so his shirt opened and the scar on his chest became visible.

The old man became very excited upon seeing the old wound. 'Wake up, wake up!' he cried.

'Look here,' he exclaimed, opening his own shirt. 'Our wounds are the same. You must be my long-lost son! I thought I would never see you again. The demon took you and your mother away.'

'This is wonderful!' said the young man.

'After all this time, I have finally found you; but what of your mother?' asked the old man. 'What happened to her? Could she still be alive?'

'I was dropped from the claws of the demon, but she was taken away in the direction of the dark mountains. I do not know where they are. She may still be there.'

'I am too frail for the journey now, my son, but you must go,' said the old man. 'I know where the dark mountains are. I will make you a map.'

They went to his house and prepared for this new journey. Soon, the young man and the raven were on their way once more.

They eventually reached the dark mountains far off to the west. After climbing to the top, they reached a large, dark cave. They entered and found a high brick wall at the back of the cave. There was a small window in the wall through which flickering lights could be seen.

'Is anyone there?' called out the young man.

'Yes,' replied a voice. A beautiful young woman came to the window. 'I am Princess Eltisha. There are a great many people here, all held prisoner by the dreadful demon. The demon has flown away in search of more people to capture, but it could return at any time. You must escape while you can. Go now!'

'No, I will not go yet,' said the young man. 'Is my mother with you? Her name is Qualetania.'

'Yes, indeed. Qualetania is here,' replied the princess.

Hearing her name mentioned, Qualetania rushed over to the window. She was overjoyed to learn that her son still alive but distressed to see him in the cave.

'Go quickly – you must leave us and save yourself!' she insisted.

Eltisha suddenly called out, 'I can hear his wings flapping. He is not far off. Quick – hide in the little tunnel here to the side.'

The young man duly concealed himself in the tunnel.

With a dreadful roar, the demon arrived back in the cave, clutching two more people in its claws. The demon pushed them through a small door in the wall and turned around.

The raven had not managed to reach the tunnel in time. It tried to sneak in but was spotted by the demon, which then noticed the young man and roared at him. 'What is this? Someone dares to come into my cave. Well, you can join the others behind the wall.'

The raven, which had never spoken before, suddenly called out, 'The mirror, the mirror! Show him his image in the mirror.'

The young man took out the fragment of mirror and pointed it at the demon. The demon was so shocked to see the ugliness of its heart reflected back at it that it screamed out in surprise. The scream was so loud and intense that the brick wall started to crumble with the reverberations. When the demon saw the wall falling, it screamed even louder and the whole wall collapsed on it, killing it. One of the bricks also landed on the raven, leaving it lying injured on the ground.

The young man came out of the tunnel, saw that the demon was dead and then went over and picked up the raven. 'Poor raven – you have been a perfect companion on my journeys. Come, I will heal your wounds.'

'Alas, no,' said the raven in a very weak voice. 'I have been gravely wounded and will soon die. Do not grieve for me, however – I have undertaken the task given to me and I can die in peace.' With that, the raven's head dropped down and he died.

Now that the wall had collapsed, all the prisoners were free. The young man was reunited with his mother. Princess Eltisha led the people down from the dark mountains to a castle where her parents, the king and queen, lived. Overjoyed to see so many of his subjects who had been thought lost, the king hosted a huge banquet in their honour. The king agreed that Princess Eltisha and the young man, who had fallen in love, could marry. They had the grandest wedding ever known in the land. The celebrations went on for many days and nights. The young man became a prince and lived in the castle with Eltisha, while his mother, Qualetania, and his father had a splendid house built near the castle; and everybody lived happily ever after.

Index

Made in the USA
Monee, IL
14 September 2026

63176224R20092